HIGH-PERFORMANCE NUTRITION FOR MASTERS ATHLETES

Lauren A. Antonucci
MS, RDN, CSSD, CDE, CDN

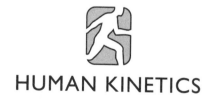

HUMAN KINETICS

Library of Congress Cataloging-in-Publication Data

Names: Antonucci, Lauren A., 1974- author.

Title: High-performance nutrition for masters athletes / Lauren A. Antonucci.

Description: Champaign : Human Kinetics, 2022. | Includes bibliographical references and index.

Identifiers: LCCN 2020043105 (print) | LCCN 2020043106 (ebook) | ISBN 9781492592976 (paperback) | ISBN 9781492592983 (epub) | ISBN 9781492592990 (pdf)

Subjects: LCSH: Athletes--Nutrition. | Cooking.

Classification: LCC TX361.A8 A58 2022 (print) | LCC TX361.A8 (ebook) | DDC 613.7/11--dc23

LC record available at https://lccn.loc.gov/2020043105

LC ebook record available at https://lccn.loc.gov/2020043106

ISBN: 978-1-4925-9297-6 (print)

This publication is written and published to provide accurate and authoritative information relevant to the subject matter presented. It is published and sold with the understanding that the author and publisher are not engaged in rendering legal, medical, or other professional services by reason of their authorship or publication of this work. If medical or other expert assistance is required, the services of a competent professional person should be sought.

The web addresses cited in this text were current as of September 2020, unless otherwise noted.

Senior Acquisitions Editor: Michelle Maloney; **Senior Developmental Editor:** Cynthia McEntire; **Managing Editors:** Shawn Donnelly and Hannah Werner; **Copyeditor**: Marissa Wold Uhrina; **Indexer:** Dan Connolly; **Permissions Manager:** Dalene Reeder; **Graphic Designers:** Denise Lowry and Sean Roosevelt; **Director, Cover Design:** Keri Evans; **Cover Designer:** Julie L. Denzer; **Cover Design Specialist:** Susan Rothermel Allen; **Photographs (cover):** adamkaz/E+/Getty Images (cyclist), Mark Ryan Pfeffer (runner); **Photographs (interior):** © Human Kinetics, unless otherwise noted; **Photo Asset Manager:** Laura Fitch; **Photo Production Manager:** Jason Allen; **Senior Art Manager:** Kelly Hendren; **Illustrations:** © Human Kinetics, unless otherwise noted; **Printer:** The P.A. Hutchison Company

Human Kinetics books are available at special discounts for bulk purchase. Special editions or book excerpts can also be created to specification. For details, contact the Special Sales Manager at Human Kinetics.

Printed in the United States of America   10 9 8 7 6 5 4 3 2 1

The paper in this book is certified under a sustainable forestry program.

Human Kinetics
1607 N. Market Street
Champaign, IL 61820
USA

United States and International
Website: **US.HumanKinetics.com**
Email: info@hkusa.com
Phone: 1-800-747-4457

Canada
Website: **Canada.HumanKinetics.com**
Email: info@hkcanada.com

E7906

In gratitude to the people in my life who have and continue to support me in all of my pursuits: my parents Peri and Mickey Wallack; my husband Russ; our children Cooper, Ryder, and Mia; my sister Rachel Wallack Cooperman; my spirit sister Nicole SinQuee; and lifelong friends Michelle Taylor, Elyse Cohen, Elisa MacPherson, Sarah Kavanagh, and Stephanie Galinkin. It is because of your support that this book and all of my other accomplishments have been possible.

CONTENTS

PREFACE

When I stood at the line for my very first running race at the age of 8, I was understandably nervous. All I could think about was going out fast, staying strong as I ran all the way around the track, winning one of the trophies I could see sitting on a table beside the track, and making my parents proud as they cheered and supported me from the sidelines.

I already knew that I loved running. My parents said I had a natural inclination and that I spent most days of my early childhood running up and down our block, driveway, or backyard while my mom followed to ensure I was safe. I had already tried (and retired from) soccer, karate, and ballet, each requiring more coordination or patience than I seemed to possess. This 400-meter neighborhood charity race was my first chance to see what I really had in terms of drive, talent, and grit. I have no recollection of what I ate for breakfast my first race morning, although I'd venture a guess it was either Cheerios or Rice Krispies, the two staple cereals we had growing up. At that time, I had no idea how important running or nutrition would become in my life, the opportunities both would provide me, the lifelong friendships I would forge, and how these two would together help shape my character and life trajectory. I also had never heard of Masters athletes, and even if I had, I would not yet have been old enough to comprehend that I would ever become one, let alone an expert writing an entire book about them.

Over three decades after my first entry into the running and racing world, I am delighted to say that I am a Masters athlete! I have spent the past 20 years of my professional career researching every sport nutrition topic as it emerged, working with athletes of all ages and abilities, and amassing as much scientific and professional nutrition information as humanly possible. I have now spent the past year putting it all together for you in this book.

Throughout middle school, high school, and college, I ran cross country and indoor and spring track, and I gobbled up the articles in each month's *Runner's World* magazine (the only source for running and nutrition information back in those days). With no internet and no home computer, magazines and anecdotes from my running coaches were where I turned for the information I craved—namely, how I could become a stronger and faster runner. I learned about fueling up with carbs, and pasta became the family ritual meal every Friday night for *years*. (Sorry, Mom, Dad, and Sis!) I read that bananas were a great source of potassium, which is key for muscle contraction, and subsequently insisted on eating one before every race. I trained hard, had a blast, and ate way more pasta, bananas, and PowerBars than I care to count. I ran really well my first three years on the varsity track team and even made it to the state meet in the 1,500 meter during the spring of ninth grade. (For some strange reason I will never understand, the boys ran a mile and we girls ran the 1,500, as if the final 100 meters were going to do us in.) I continued to run well but was also injured off and on from 10th grade through college. During that time I spent countless hours icing various body parts, was prescribed orthotics when my knees started to hurt, went through several rounds of physical therapy for various injuries, and visited a chiropractor when my lower back was troubling me. On my own, I sought to learn everything I could about both physiology and nutrition, and I was fascinated by the answers I found.

In college I contemplated pursuing sports medicine, athletic training, and physical therapy as career options; served as a trainer for our college basketball team, a research assistant in a lab studying Alzheimer's disease, and a smoking cessation research lab assistant; and graduated with a BS in psychobiology. Throughout those four years, it had become clear to me that nutrition and hydration played a major role in both short- and long-term health and athletic performance, and I had determined that learning about and helping others to implement the latest scientific discoveries for both mind and body were what I wanted to spend my life doing. I had known several teammates and friends who struggled with eating disorders and other athletes who didn't seem to give a second thought to how they fueled their bodies.

I applied to several graduate schools around the country and was thrilled when I received a scholarship to study nutritional biochemistry at the University of California at Berkeley! There, I had the honor of working in laboratories studying gluconeogenesis, muscle metabolism, and respiratory oxygen exchange, three topics I continue to study today. From some of the best and brightest minds I'll ever meet, I learned about how we use, digest, and process food. What struck me most during my time at Berkeley was the practice of continually asking difficult questions, working tirelessly to uncover important answers, and never taking any one piece of research or fact for granted or as the final answer.

Thereafter, I returned to New York City and completed a master's degree in clinical nutrition from New York University while working as a personal trainer at Equinox Health Club and simultaneously training for my first Half Ironman Triathlon (now called Ironman 70.3) with the Leukemia and Lymphoma Society's Team in Training program. I immersed myself in nutrition, training, and physiology, and I couldn't get enough.

My interest in sport nutrition really flourished in college and strengthened when I ran my first marathon my senior year, when I did not yet know that I should have had a nutrition plan. I simply sucked down a few energy gels and attempted to bite into frozen granola bars while training in freezing upstate New York. Next, while at Berkeley for graduate school, I ran several mountain trail races and then the Sacramento Marathon, which is when I experienced firsthand what it feels like to bonk. I was well trained and felt fine . . . until I wasn't. Somewhere around mile 18, my legs locked up and felt like cement, and my vision started to blur. Luckily, I was near an aid station. I stopped, took in two cups of sport drinks and an energy gel, walked for a few minutes, and was able to finish safely. It was this experience that solidified my dream to both continue to push my body's limits in long-course running and triathlons, and to fuel myself and other athletes to be their best in their pursuits.

I started experimenting further with my own fueling while completing 8- to 10-hour training blocks as I prepared for my first Ironman Distance Triathlon, Ironman Lake Placid, which I completed with my then-boyfriend, now husband, in 2001. We drank Ensure, made peanut butter and jelly sandwiches, and taste-tested each new gel and sport drink brand and flavor as it emerged.

When our first son, Cooper, was born in March 2006, I quickly went from training to compete to accepting that running to and from work was going to be my training, and that running while pushing a baby jogger was not only acceptable but enjoyable. This also meant nutritional changes, because up until this point I had always been an early-morning runner. Now there was nursing, pumping, and more to be done before I could head out for my run-fix. Being a glass-half-full kind of person, I looked at the upside and appreciated the freedom I gained in being able to run with my child (once he was six months old and able to be pushed in a baby jogger) as well as the arm strength I was building pushing him around Central Park without setting foot in a weight room.

I researched nutrition for nursing and athletic moms and disappointingly found very little definitive information. As my nutrition practice in New York City took off and work life got busier, I prioritized time to resume strength training (very early in the morning, before Cooper awoke) over cleaning the apartment most days, because I knew that especially once I was in my 30s, I *needed* to strength train and that my apartment was never really going to be organized with a newborn. I researched how my nutritional needs might have shifted due to that training change and found some, but not enough, information to satisfy my curious scientific brain.

The way I see it, each phase of life provides an opportunity to re-evaluate our training, nutrition, and lifestyle choices. Each new decade, career change, birth of a child, or registration for a new team or race provides an opportunity to look inward, not only for the strength and energy to make it through, but also to figure out how to be our best selves and live our best lives. I have personally done a great deal of shifting in my training, nutrition, and lifestyle priorities over the past 20-plus years as I went to college, completed two graduate programs, worked as a clinical dietitian at New York Presbyterian Hospital for several years, got married, started my own private nutrition practice, gave birth to our three children, and am raising a family with my husband. This constant shifting is something I am sure many of you can relate to, and it can either help us keep our priorities in check and enable us to adapt to life's curves, or it can throw us for a loop. Along with each major life change, I have reassessed how my needs shifted from both physiological and lifestyle perspectives, and I adjusted my training and nutrition to match. I looked for scientific answers to confirm these shifts and to learn what was important in terms of fueling athletes in each decade of life, and was never satisfied with the scant information I was able to find. After more than 20 years of working with athletes of all ages and abilities and of reading all available scientific information about our changing nutritional needs as we age, I jumped at the chance to write this book.

This book is for people who consider themselves a Masters athlete, which means every athlete over the age of 35, or who are Masters just getting started in physical fitness for the first time and want to continue to be an athlete throughout their lives. This book is also intended to be a tool for coaches, dietitians, strength and conditioning professionals, medical doctors, and trainers who work with Masters athletes and want the latest research put into practical terms. My goal in writing *High-Performance Nutrition for Masters Athletes* is that the research and interviews of professionals, coaching, and athletes will provide all the answers you are looking for—and many you didn't even realize you needed to know—all in this one book.

If we really pay attention, we realize that our bodies crave movement as well as a varied and well-rounded assortment of foods and food groups. Certainly, each of us has our go-to activities and favorite foods, but these preferences generally do not take into account our changing needs as we age. As creatures of habit, we often do and eat the same things day after day and year after year. Personally, if I weren't paying attention, I would likely end up running, running, and running some more, plus repeating the same sequence of strength training moves I've been doing since I was 18, while eating meal after meal of oatmeal, almond nut butter and banana sandwiches, fish tacos, and ice cream. When we continually (albeit often unintentionally) neglect some necessary aspects of training and nutrition by engaging in the same activities and eating the same foods over and over again, we increase our chances of deficiencies in one area and excesses in another. We then spend an inordinate amount of time trying to analyze where we went wrong when we feel overtrained, tired, or injured. By learning about our physiology and changing nutritional needs, and then adapting our training and eating to meet us where we are, we can continue to engage in our sport for a lifetime.

In part I, I define the Masters athlete across sports and outline the many athletic opportunities we continue to have as we age. I also discuss the many negative effects that lack of physical activity and poor nutritional choices have on our health (as individuals and in our aging society as a whole) and what you can do to maintain your vitality, energy, health, and performance.

Part I also includes the latest scientific research intertwined with practical advice and interviews with medical professionals, exercise physiologists, and athletes. This helps explain how both our physiology and nutritional needs change as we move through the decades of our lives. I debunk myths behind some arbitrary guidelines and also address expected changes in resting metabolic rate, $\dot{V}O_2$max, and body fat percentage as we age. I then teach you the nutrition and training tricks you need to know in order to remain at your peak. I include nutritional guidelines for athletes with medical concerns such as high blood pressure, cardiovascular disease, and diabetes. Food truly is medicine, and we should use that knowledge to our advantage.

Part II is all about fueling and the changing nutritional needs of Masters athletes. I explain the importance of all macronutrients—carbohydrate, protein, and fat—for all athletes and their needs for each by sport and age range. You also learn about the vitamins and minerals most adults lack as well as what you can do about it. I include essential information on your changing needs for calcium, B-vitamins, iron, and omega-3, all of which are critical to your health and athletic performance.

Because Masters athletes are at increased risk of dehydration, I explain how to conduct sweat testing on your own to help you determine, then meet, your individual hydration needs, and I lead you through everything you need to know about your changing fluid and hydration needs.

Part II concludes with the important topic of underfueling in sport and the toll unhealthy or restrictive eating behaviors take on mental and physical health and performance. We discuss the prevalence, challenges, real-life examples, and successes in overcoming eating disorders and disordered eating in athletes and the slippery slope of underfueling in athletes. We review how to recognize eating disorders in athletes, consequences of long-term reduced energy availability, and possible treatments for athletes with eating disorders.

Part III brings us into the nitty gritty of fueling our competitions and long-term performance as Masters athletes. I walk you through calculating your preworkout nutritional needs based on your sport, and I delineate what you need to take in during training, racing, and competing based on duration, intensity, and type of activity. Lastly, you learn the real truth about your recovery nutrition needs and how to consistently meet them and prolong your life as an athlete. I have created simple charts to help you determine your pre-, during-, and postworkout nutritional needs, and I have included sample meal plans to show you how to put it all together. Think of this book as your own customizable adventure in resetting your eating habits to fully meet your needs as the Masters athlete that you are.

Scattered throughout each chapter is the opportunity to learn from real-life examples. I have interviewed and recounted the stories of many amazing athletes who have been at the top of their game since before becoming a Masters athlete and who still maintain top physical conditioning. You get an inside peek into how they changed their nutrition and training regimes to stay at their best from age 35 and beyond, or how they wish they had done so sooner. I know you will appreciate hearing about and learning from their journeys.

Thank you for embarking on this journey with me in exploring your changing nutritional needs as Masters athletes. I hope you enjoy reading and digesting the information as much as I have enjoyed writing it for you.

Yours in health and motion for life.

—Lauren

ACKNOWLEDGMENTS

It is with great sincerity and much appreciation that I thank each of the 26 amazing athletes who so graciously allowed me to interview them and to share their stories with you in my book:

- Kathrine Switzer (kathrineswitzer.com)
- Pete Fleury
- Polly de Mille
- Jonathan Cane (Instagram @citycoachms and @coachcane)
- Keith LaScalea
- Tony Claudino
- Meb Keflezighi (marathonmeb.com)
- Norman Goluskin (ngoluskin@hotmail.com)
- Gordon Bakoulis
- Sarah True (Instagram @Sarah.b.true, Twitter @sgroffy, Facebook @ SarahTrue)
- Ben Kessel (priorityfitnesstraining.com, Instagram @priorityfitness)
- Ryan Hall (Instagram @Ryanhall3)
- Kara Goucher (karagoucher.com; Instagram, Facebook, and Twitter @ Karagoucher; and @cleansportco on Instagram)
- Erica Agran (Instagram @Ericaagran, Facebook @Ericafinds)
- Jackie Edwards Flowers
- Connor Barwin (Instagram @connorbarwin98; Make the World Better (MTWB) Foundation, MTWB.org)
- Meghan Newcomer (Instagram @meghannewcomer, beencouraged-bymeghan.com)
- Gail Waesche Kislevitz
- Stephanie Roth Goldberg (intuitivepsychotherapynyc.com, Instagram @embodiedpsychotherapist)
- Ellen Hart (Instagram @ellenhart58)
- Roger Robinson (roger-robinson.com)
- Stephen England (Instagram @rundiabetes)
- B.J. (Bedford) Miller
- Deena Kastor (Instagram @Deena8050, Twitter @DeenaKastor)

- Ramon Bermo (Instagram and Facebook @Ramonbermo, https://www. cancer.org/involved/fundraise/determination.html)
- Paul Thompson (Instagram @holmfirthharrier)

Each of these conversations was inspiring and these are interactions that I will never forget. The accounts of their athletic and nutritional journeys were insightful, honest, and very powerful. I hope you enjoyed reading each of their stories as much as I enjoyed writing them.

I would like to thank my parents Peri and Mickey Wallack, to whom I am forever grateful, for encouraging me to try anything and everything I was interested in, never once telling me I couldn't do something because I am a girl or woman, too short, not good enough, or not smart enough, and for cheering me on at hundreds of swimming and track meets. You supported me through all my decisions (the good, the bad, and the sometimes ugly), and for that I am thankful. My dad showed me the importance of working hard and never missed a day of work, but once home, he was ready to play and taught me the importance of being silly and not taking myself too seriously. He never complained, not even when he spent the last year of his life sick with cancer, in and out of treatments, surgeries, and hospital visits. He loved deeply, and I miss him daily. My mom always spoke to my sister and me like adults, explained things in real terms, and continues to show us by example that women can do anything and should be respected and taken seriously. She taught us to never let anyone take advantage of us and to advocate politely, but firmly, for our ideals. Together they taught us to work hard, to be good and kind, to respect and think kindly of others, and to follow our dreams.

I thank my husband Russ, who I met in a bike shop (our children love this story), and who leads me bravely and boldly on adventures near and far, from France to Turkey, Costa Rica to Cambodia, and across the United States, usually with outdoor adventures or races in mind. I thank you for supporting me in all my pursuits, from leaving a steady job to start my own private practice just after our honeymoon in 2003, to excitedly agreeing to my registering and training for the Escape From Alcatraz triathlon in 2019 after not racing in years, to supporting me in writing this book without hesitation, even though we already had a lot on our plate, because you could hear my excitement in tackling this new project. For all of this, and for being my computer technician, bike mechanic, idea guy, and navigator, I love and appreciate you, and am here to support you.

Our three amazing children inspire me every day to be a better person, to slow down and appreciate the little things, to be present more, to listen closely, and to love more deeply than I ever thought possible. Cooper, your sense of direction and determination have been evident from a very young age as you climbed higher, jumped farther, and read sooner than I thought any child could. You inspire me to continue to reach for the stars. You continually show me what is possible when you have a big goal worth working

WHO Key Facts for a Healthy Diet

- Energy intake should be in balance with energy expenditure.
- Limit free sugar intake to less than 10 percent of total energy intake (12 tsp, 59 mL) per day.
- Fat intake should be less than 30 percent of total energy intake per day.
- Choose unsaturated fats such as fish, avocado, and nuts, and sunflower, soybean, canola, and olive oils.
- Limit saturated fat from sources such as fatty meat, butter, palm and coconut oils, cream, cheese, ghee, and lard to less than 10 percent of total energy intake per day.
- Limit the intake of trans fat, often found in commercially prepared and packaged baked goods and fried foods, to less than 1 percent of total energy intake per day.
- Limit salt intake to less than 5 grams per day (sodium intake to <2 g per day).
- Include plenty of fresh fruits, vegetables, legumes (lentils, beans), nuts, and whole grains.
- Consume at least 5 portions or servings of fruits and vegetables each day (500 g).

Following the plethora of research that shows how eating a diet rich in fruits and vegetables can help lower chronic disease risk, improve preexisting health conditions, and aid in weight management, the WHO also recommends that governments create national nutrition and agriculture policies and incentives that increase investments in the growth, trade, production, and consumption of healthy foods, including fruits and vegetables. The WHO calls for decreased incentives for both producers and retailers to make and sell foods that are high in sodium, saturated and trans fats, and added sugars. They also advocate for such policies on both a national and local level.

To some these goals may seem lofty, while to others they may already be a part of your daily life. Sadly, for the United States as a whole during the decade spanning 1994 to 2005, overall mean fruit and vegetable consumption actually *decreased* slightly (Blanck et al. 2008). Only 1 in 10 American adults meet the federal guidelines for intake of fruits and vegetables (U.S. Department of Health and Human Services 2017). No wonder we can't control our rates of chronic disease.

The Dietary Guidelines for Americans are revised every five years based on a thorough review of the scientific literature on diet, nutrition health promotion, and disease prevention. The 2015-2020 version is in line with the WHO recommendations above and sets intake goals of 1.5 to 2 cups of whole fruit daily and 2 to 3 cups of vegetables daily, and emphasizes the need for an overall increase in fruit and vegetable intake in order to decrease risk of diet-related chronic diseases including type 2 diabetes, some cancers, obesity, and heart diseases (Dietary Guidelines Advisory Committee 2015).

Sadly, but not surprisingly, dietary habits in the United States and around the world do not align with national or global nutritional recommendations. Approximately 9 in 10 Americans are consistently low in intake of both total vegetables and total fruits, and most Americans consume more added sugar, saturated fat, and sodium than is optimal for health (Dietary Guidelines Advisory Committee 2015). Additionally, the daily caloric intake of many is higher than necessary for their individual age and activity level, resulting in over two thirds of all U.S. adults (and almost one third of all U.S. children) considered either overweight or obese.

Spotlight on Pete Fleury

Pete Fleury is an amazing runner, science teacher, and coach who has inspired count-less young runners though his coaching and as a lifelong runner. He has been running for more than 40 years, has run 43 marathons (2:49 PR) and many ultramarathons, and remains active each day. His first marathon (the Long Island Marathon) was in 1979, and his last (the New York City) was in 2006, which he ran to celebrate his 60th birthday.

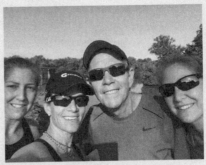

Courtesy of Lauren Antonucci.

What is your approach as a Masters athlete?

I know people who log every mile and everything they eat—to me that is a bit overboard. I don't really worry about it. I have certainly cut back on the amount I am eating some because I don't run as far or as fast, but I am more fit than most people my age. I enjoy it, and today, on my 73rd birthday (April 2019), I still feel good, and that is what is important to me.

Speaking of the benefits of exercise, I had a stress test for the second time in my life at my annual physical in December 2018. My doctor told me that I didn't need one because I was obviously fit, but I said I'd like to get one, just to be sure. They put me on a treadmill with four people watching me. I thought, Why do they need so many people in here? First they made me walk, then they elevated the treadmill. Finally, it got fast enough for me to run, and he made me hold on "for safety." I told him I didn't need to do that, but he insisted that I did. Then, and I wasn't even moving very fast yet, he told me to stop, and said it was over. He then told me that I have the heart of a 35- to 40-year-old. These results were good and I feel good, so I know I am doing something right. The test was worth it for peace of mind.

feedback loop between decreased exercise, decreased muscle mass, and decreased energy needs can be partially interrupted with optimal fueling to allow for continued intense training and maintenance of muscle mass and LBM throughout our lifetime. This is of course good news for athletes, but it also bodes well for overall health and longevity, because increased muscle mass and strength may lead to decreases in fall risk and our ability to perform activities of daily living and to prolong independence as we advance in age. For more about training Masters athletes, see the sidebar on the next page about exercise physiologist, athlete, and coach, Jonathan Cane.

Basal Metabolic Rate

I can't count the number of times I've heard someone say, "My metabolism started to tank as soon as I hit the age of [insert person's chosen age of blame here]." Is there any truth behind this statement, and if so, is there anything we can do to slow or attenuate this decrease in energy requirements as we age? Thankfully, the answer is yes. One initial study demonstrated that mean energy requirements (the amount of nutrition or total calories one needs to take in during a given day in order to maintain weight) increased by about 15 percent following a 12-week resistance training program in adults ages 56 to 80 (Campbell et al. 1994). Their work demonstrated that both resting energy expenditure (the number of calories your body requires per day when at rest) increased and energy cost of exercise (the amount of calories you burn performing a given activity) increased following resistance training. They concluded that resistance training can be an effective way to both decrease body fat mass and maintain lean muscle tissue as we age. Another promising study found increases in both basal metabolic rate (BMR) and the thermic effect of food (TEF) (Lundholm et al. 1986). TEF is the increase in energy expenditure above baseline following the ingestion of food in order to process your food for use and storage. They examined physically well-trained older men and postulated that this effect may be attributable to their increased muscle mass compared to sedentary controls.

Skin Elasticity

As we also have begun to notice, our skin loses elasticity as we age. The largest organ in our bodies, the epidermis is quite complex. It makes up 6 percent of our total body weight and provides not only protection from the outside world, but is also integrally involved in regulating our body temperature and internal hydration (see chapter 9), sensory functions, and immunological surveillance (Farage et al. 2013). Immune surveillance is the process by which our immune system is able to identify precancerous and cancerous cells and eliminate them before they are able to multiply and do us harm (Swann and Smyth 2007).

Spotlight on Jonathan Cane

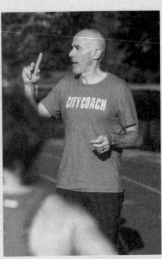

Jonathan holds a master's degree in exercise physiology and has earned certifications from ACSM, USA Cycling, and the National Strength and Conditioning Association. As a former category 3 cyclist and coach of endurance athletes for more than 25 years, Jonathan is a wealth of information on exercise physiology.

Courtesy of Zach Hetrick.

What are the major physiological changes you see in Masters athletes?

I am an exercise physiologist at heart, and also an athlete who knows that everyone, at every age, is entitled to have a bad day or a bad race. I will push my athletes hard at any age as long as they have the ability to train and recover well. Continuing to train hard (with adequate recovery nutrition and time between sessions) is the key to maintaining our $\dot{V}O_2$max, muscle mass, and strength, and preventing injuries. We need to look at the science, and we need to accurately interpret the science and train and recover accordingly . . . and then we also need to not blame everything on "age catching up with me." From both perspectives of performance and reducing injury risk, resistance training is nonnegotiable for Masters athletes.

How do you see nutrition and changing physiology interplay?

If we look at why some Masters athletes continue to thrive (instead of continually thinking about why are they falling apart) and ask why, then we can really get some-

A great deal of literature exists connecting nutrition with skin health and skin aging. (See chapter 8.) Intrinsic skin aging is a result of factors that are inherent in all body systems and are not thought to be modifiable (Tzellos et al. 2009). Extrinsic skin aging is defined as skin aging that results from external factors including the environment, sun exposure and ultraviolet (UV) irradiation, smoking, pollution, sleep deprivation, and poor nutrition (Schagen et al. 2012). Physical activity, stress reduction, and a balanced diet that includes plenty of antioxidative foods are known prevention strategies against premature skin aging. In terms of extrinsic aging, studies have concluded that adequate intakes of both vitamin C (ascorbic acid) and tocopherols (vitamin E), which are naturally occurring antioxidants that work to scavenger highly reactive free radicals, are important in maintaining skin collagen and working against aging skin (Schagen et al. 2012). Eating a diet high in vitamin C–rich foods, which includes most fresh fruits and vegetables, is a great start toward careful about getting in some protein and some carbohydrate after each workout. Years ago, I would not have been able to tell you how many vegetables I had eaten during a day—now I can. I also started using a protein powder and a curcumin supplement, and I make a much more concerted effort to foam roll and keep flexible. I am doing more of what I have always told my athletes to do.

How do you help Masters athletes?

I work with a ton of Masters athletes for performance testing, injury prevention, and postinjury recovery, so I have seen it all. Resistance training strengthens your muscles around your bones, which in turn keeps your bones in better alignment and loads your joints in better alignment and helps prevent injury. Measuring bone density is something I highly recommend—most people should be doing this earlier than they might think.

What overall words of wisdom do you have for Masters athletes?

- Choose quality over just quantity, and make sure you are balancing workouts.
- Have a purpose for each workout, and spend your time more wisely.
- Be consistent but flexible with your training so that you don't drive yourself into the ground, because if you do, you will have a much tougher time climbing out at age 50 versus 20.
- Think about how you have gotten hurt in the past and how you can avoid making the same mistakes again.
- Learn to pick up on your body's cues.
- Stay hydrated.
- Eat better.
- Start thinking about bone density (if you haven't already).
- Running may make your heart sing, while foam rolling and eating veggies may not—but they will keep you doing what you love.

Polly's Favorite Postrace Meal

Homemade cookies and fresh milk from the dairy farm at the Strafford (VT) Nordic Center Turkey Trot. Pure bliss.

Adequate sleep duration and quality are important for both athletic performance and optimal recovery. A review article by Shona L. Halson (2014) describes how inadequate sleep is known to adversely affect learning, memory, and cognition as well as pain perception, immunity, inflammation, appetite, food intake, protein synthesis, and glucose metabolism (figure 2.3), all of which potentially reduce athletic performance.

Halson's article, titled "Sleep in Elite Athletes and Nutritional Interventions to Enhance Sleep," explains that although the exact functions of sleep are not completely understood, it is generally accepted that sleep helps our bodies recover from our previous day as well as prepare for optimal functioning on subsequent days. Studies show that restricting sleep to less than six hours per night for four or more consecutive nights impairs cognitive function as well as mood. You may have also noticed that when you are not getting adequate sleep for several consecutive nights or longer, you are more likely to get sick and/or tend to consume an increased amount of total or sugary foods. Finally, studies have also demonstrated decreased cycling power with decreased sleep and a subsequent improvement in both mood and performance when sleep duration is allowed to increase again (Andrade et al. 2016).

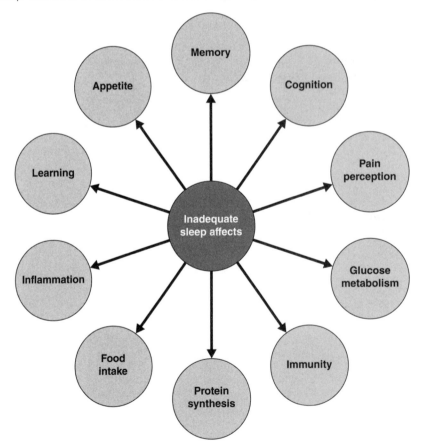

FIGURE 2.3   Negative effects of inadequate sleep on multiple body systems.

Many studies have shown a positive correlation between increased risk of obesity and diabetes in those individuals who are sleep deprived. Van Cauter et al. (2008) showed decreased brain glucose utilization, alterations in balance, increased cortisol levels, and increases in inflammatory processes that accompany sleep deprivation. Additionally, they showed that sleep deprivation leads to decreased leptin and increased ghrelin production. Leptin is a protein produced by fat cells and acts mainly in the regulation of appetite and fat storage. Ghrelin is a gut hormone that has been labeled "the hunger hormone," because it is known for its appetite- and food intake–stimulating effects as well as increased fat deposition and growth hormone release (Pradhan, Samson, and Sun 2013).

According to many research studies (e.g., Hansen et al. 2014) as well as the National Sleep Foundation (2020), certain foods improve sleep duration and quality.

- *Milk* contains tryptophan, melatonin, calcium, and magnesium, all of which have been linked with improved sleep. Some people have made a link between the childhood ritual of enjoying a glass of milk before bed and good sleep.

- *Lean proteins*, including the infamous sleep inducer, turkey, can also help facilitate a good night's sleep due to their tryptophan content.

- *Nuts*, especially walnuts and almonds, are high in naturally occurring tryptophan and melatonin.

- *Fruits,* including kiwi, whole cherries, tart cherry juice, bananas, pineapple, raspberries, and oranges, all contain melatonin, which may help you fall asleep faster and stay asleep throughout the night.

- A cup of *caffeine-free tea* can be a good source of calming herbs such as chamomile, passionflower, and valerian plus L-theanine, which can promote a feeling of calm. Enjoying a cup of tea before bed also is a great psychological ritual.

- *Fatty fish* and other sources of both vitamin D and omega-3 fatty acids may help regulate serotonin and allow for adequate sleep. Hansen et al. (2014) found that consuming fatty fish three times a week for six months (instead of chicken, pork, or beef consumed in the control group) improved vitamin D and omega-3 fatty acid concentrations and leads to decreased wake time during sleep and decreased time to fall asleep, or sleep latency. However, after looking at the results of several studies, it is difficult to say whether it is the increased intake of fatty fish and improved vitamin D status that improves sleep, or that the consumption of other meat consumption (chicken, pork, or beef) worsens sleep quality. Clearly, more research is needed in this area.

Connections Among Sleep, Menopause, and Nutrition

The years during which hormonal changes begin that lead to cessation of menstruation in women result in a slew of physiological and metabolic changes that may warrant alterations in previous nutritional intake. According to the National Sleep Foundation (2019), women experience more sleep disturbances during the time of perimenopause, during which less estrogen and progesterone are produced. They report an increase in insomnia of up to 50 to 60 percent among menopausal and postmenopausal women versus just 15 percent reporting sleep disturbances before this hormonal shift begins. Of postmenopausal woman with high BMI 47 percent report sleep apnea (up from 21% premenopause). Many women also report difficulty falling asleep or staying asleep, mood swings, and hot flashes once perimenopause begins.

In addition to the usual healthy sleep hygiene habits we should all adopt, including setting aside down time before bed, postmenopausal women are advised to avoid large meals or spicy and acidic foods before bed and to reduce their intake of caffeine and alcohol in order to reduce hot flashes, which are counterproductive to getting a good night's sleep. Women may also want to include whole soy foods that contain natural phytoestrogens, plant hormones similar to estrogen, which have been shown to help decrease hot flashes. Eating an overall healthy and balanced diet becomes more important than ever, as can getting adequate calcium and vitamin D in order to prevent and treat osteoporosis.

In chapter 3 we will continue to explore expected changes with aging but from a more medical perspective. We will delve into expected but unwanted increases in blood pressure, cholesterol, insulin resistance, obesity, and some cancers, as well as how your training and nutrition can reduce your risk and improve your outcomes.

3 | Nutritional Strategies to Manage and Prevent Disease

As we age, we can expect decreases in average $\dot{V}O_2$max, muscle mass/lean body mass, movement, and function (ACSM et al. 2009). Additionally, we see increased incidence of many chronic diseases. The good news is that exercise consistency tends to decrease the risk of chronic diseases such as cardiovascular disease (CVD), diabetes, obesity, some cancers, osteopenia, arthritis, and sarcopenia, which otherwise increase with each decade of life. The silver lining for Masters athletes is that even moderately fit adults have consistently shown decreased risk of CVD and overall mortality verses sedentary individuals. Consistent exercise has been shown to decrease LDL (the bad cholesterol), increase HDL (the good cholesterol) and decrease overall triglycerides.

This chapter looks at the consistent nutrition principles that can help vastly reduce our risk of developing most of the major chronic diseases that plague the Western world. Rates of heart disease, hypertension, diabetes, and many types of cancer are extremely high in the United States, but sound nutrition practices, along with an active lifestyle, will help reduce your chances of developing these chronic health conditions or improve your overall health outcomes if you already have or ever develop a chronic medical condition.

The Academy of Nutrition and Dietetics (AND) recommends eating foods from a wide variety of food groups, including fruits, vegetables, whole grains, low-fat or fat-free dairy, lean meat, poultry, fish, beans, eggs, and nuts, and following an overall eating pattern that is low in saturated and trans fats, salt, and added sugars. AND also recommends plenty of dark green and orange fruits and vegetables, varied proteins, and more than 3 ounces of whole grains daily. They advise eating more mono- and unsaturated fats and low-fat dairy with added vitamin D. They also explain that omega-3, polyunsaturated fats may help with brain and nervous system function and decrease cholesterol levels and overall inflammation, and as such should be included in greater quantity than other fats.

I have my own way of explaining healthy and balanced eating to clients (as well as friends, family members, and our children) that seems to really resonate with people. I make an analogy between eating and getting dressed. Bear with me for a minute and this just might make more sense of eating than you ever thought possible. We all get dressed each and every day, right? And on the most basic level, and from a very early age, we know what to do: choose a shirt, underwear, pants (or shorts or skirt), socks . . . you get the idea. Well, what if we thought of choosing foods for meals or snacks in the same way. There are no *good* or *bad* foods. There are foods you are in the mood to eat today, and others you are not. Just as you can choose whichever color shirt suits your mood on any given day, and whether you need a tank top or a sweater based on the weather, you can select whichever foods you are in the mood for and adjust to your hunger. You can think of each food category (for this analogy, I differentiate them as carbs, protein, fats, and veg) as a different category of clothing. Then, choose what you are in the mood for, and be sure you cover all of your bases (you wouldn't go outside for a run without your shorts would you? Or to a work meeting without a shirt and shoes?). One morning, you might be in the mood for a bagel (carb), and add egg (protein), avocado (fat), and tomato (veg!). You made what you want, you covered your bases, and you then enjoy however much you are hungry for. Later, you might be in the mood for rice or potatoes (carb), and pair it with tofu (protein), peanut sauce (fat), and carrots and mushrooms (veg). The main idea here, and where freedom from food rules comes in, is that you are always in the driver's seat in terms of choosing *and eating* whichever foods you really want. Of course, not all meals will contain all food groups, and we could make analogies for that too (choose a dress or jumpsuit and you don't need another bottom). I hope you can use this silly but practical analogy as a tool in helping you navigate your nutritional needs while remembering that all foods are *allowed* and can fit into a healthy athlete's diet and life.

Down and Dirty Facts About Fats

When you read the words *dietary fat*, you may think of butter or avocados, or of cholesterol and triglyceride levels—or you may immediately become confused—which fats "should" we eat? In my nutrition practice, I see athletes of all ages and abilities who are unsure of which fats to eat more of and how much is too much. It may be helpful to define terms related to fats.

Triglycerides are fats obtained from foods we eat, including butter, margarine, and other oils. Excess calories and sugars from alcohol, refined sugars, and sodas are also converted into triglycerides in our body, carried around in our circulatory system, and eventually stored.

Cholesterol is not actually a fat but is a waxy substance that can both be made by our liver and ingested in animal products. Our livers produce cholesterol, because it is an essential component of our nerves and cell walls and is integral for both hormone production and digestion. That means that cholesterol is not just an enemy, but also a necessary friend. Of course, problems occur when too much cholesterol is either produced by the liver or ingested in animal foods, and because excess cholesterol and triglycerides are continually carried around in our blood, this can lead to increased risk of heart disease.

The good news is that exercise can be helpful in terms of using and helping to clear triglycerides and cholesterol from the blood, but unfortunately, it does not act as a singular fountain of youth. The nutritional choices we make day in day out, and year after year, play an integral role in how, and how quickly, we age and how our genetics play out in terms of chronic diseases.

Omega-3, polyunsaturated fats, including ALA, DHA, and EPA, cannot be made by our bodies and therefore need to be ingested. Good sources of omega-3 fats include salmon, herring, sardines, lake trout, and Atlantic or Pacific mackerel as well as walnuts, flaxseeds, chia seeds, hemp seeds, and some eggs. AND recommends eating fatty fish two times per week.

Monounsaturated fats, which include olive, canola, peanut, sesame, and safflower oils as well as avocado, peanut butter, and most nuts and seeds, have been shown to increase HDL (often referred to as "good" cholesterol) and help decrease LDL (often referred to as "bad" cholesterol). Swapping out saturated fats, including butter and lard, for mono- or polyunsaturated fats may help decrease total cholesterol and keep the arteries clear. We will delve deeply into the importance of adequate dietary fat intake in chapter 7.

Preventing and Managing Diabetes Through Diet

Diabetes currently affects more than 30 million Americans, or 1 in 10 adults in the United States, according to the American Diabetes Association (2018). Approximately 90 percent of people with diabetes have type 2 diabetes, while the other 10 percent have type 1 diabetes. Each year in the United States 1.5 million new cases are diagnosed. In addition, a whopping 7.3 million people are thought to have undiagnosed diabetes. Overall, diabetes is said to cost more than $327 billion annually—$237 billion in direct medical costs and the rest in lost labor. According to a recent review, among all people who have diabetes, 20.9 percent are said to have it under good control, while 45.2 percent are treated but not well controlled, 9.2 percent are aware they have diabetes but are not being treated, and 24.7 percent are not yet aware they have it. For a good summary of diabetes, see the article "What is Diabetes?" at the Centers for Disease Control website (CDC 2019a).

Type 1 diabetes (DM1) is an autoimmune reaction in which the body attacks the cells in the pancreas until the pancreas cannot make much, or any, insulin. Since insulin is required by the body to enable sugar to enter cells to be used for energy and to stabilize blood sugar, people with DM1 need to take insulin through multiple daily injections or by using an insulin pump. Important aspects of controlling diabetes include closely counting carbohydrate intake and taking insulin to match that intake; monitoring blood pressure, cholesterol, and other health parameters; and being physically active.

Type 2 diabetes (DM2) is a result of our cells failing to respond adequately to the insulin produced by the pancreas, also known as insulin resistance. Insulin resistance is thought to occur when the cells can no longer respond normally to insulin. Over time, the pancreas tries to up-regulate insulin production but eventually cannot keep up, and blood sugar begins to rise. Prolonged high blood sugar leads to increased incidence of such issues as heart disease, vision problems, and kidney disease. Signs and symptoms of both types of diabetes include excessive thirst, increased urination, unintentional weight loss, blurry vision, slowed wound heading, and increased infections. Most people with DM2 are diagnosed after age 45. However, the incidence of youth and children diagnosed with DM2 has unfortunately been on the rise.

The good news for Masters athletes, with or without diabetes, is that athletes are more insulin sensitive than sedentary people regardless of age. This is especially important for Masters athletes since insulin resistance tends to worsen as we age (Amati et al. 2009).

Controlling one's blood glucose level is a primary goal in diabetes management. For those with type 2 diabetes, this generally involves learning about the carbohydrate content of foods, keeping carbohydrate intake both moderate and consistent (in terms of timing and amount eaten) from day to day, and consistently taking the medication prescribed by their MD. For those with type 1 diabetes, blood sugar management also involves learning the carbohydrate content of all foods, and then understanding how much insulin to take (either by injection or through an insulin pump) in order to cover both their basal needs and the carbohydrate eaten. As a certified diabetes educator, I work with athletes who have diabetes to help them ensure both adequate nutritional intake and to keep their blood sugars within normal range during their daily lives and while engaging in exercise. Choosing more nutrient-dense, slowly digested, whole-grain carbohydrate such as beans, lentils, and oats as well as whole fruits, vegetables, and whole-grain breads is a cornerstone of my diabetes education with both athletes and nonathletes.

A starting point for teaching nutrition for blood sugar management is to fill half the plate with nonstarchy vegetables, a quarter of the plate with lean protein, and a quarter of the plate with grains, carbs, or starch. Lean proteins include fish, lean poultry and meat, eggs, beans, low-fat dairy (especially higher protein, Greek-style yogurts), and tofu. Nonstarchy veggies include everything from tomatoes to broccoli to spinach, but not potatoes, peas, and corn, which are considered carbohydrates due to their higher carb content. One important note is that athletes with and without diabetes will often need more carbohydrate than a quarter of the plate due to high calorie and high carbohydrate needs to fuel their activity and recovery. So with diabetes, as with many medical conditions, you need to balance your medical needs with your needs as an athlete—and I am here to help you do just that.

Finally, *everyone* can enjoy sweets in moderation. Individuals who have diabetes generally find they have better blood sugar control when they eat sweets along with a meal or with other foods that contain lean protein, fiber, and good fats to minimize impact on postprandial (postmeal) blood sugar, and should always pay attention to how eating different foods affects their blood sugar. There is no such thing as the perfect or ideal carbohydrate for people with diabetes or for athletes, which we will discuss in later chapters of this book.

In terms of dietary fat intake, eating less saturated fat and trans fat (avoiding hydrogenated and partially hydrogenated oils and deep-fried foods) and increasing intake of healthier mono- and polyunsaturated oils such as olive, peanut, avocado, canola (oils that are liquid at room temperature), plus flax, nuts, avocados, and seeds are recommended for people with diabetes, just as it is for those with heart disease, which is more prevalent in people with diabetes. Following this Mediterranean style of eating has been shown to help improve blood sugar levels as well as reduce rates of heart disease (Mozaffarian et al. 2011). Eating 20 to 35 grams of fiber per day is also recommended; this helps with satiety, blood sugar control, and heart health. A continual theme in nutrition for overall health and disease risk reduction is that increased intake of total dietary fiber is associated with decreases in all-cause mortality and is a cornerstone of our nutrition recommendations for most individuals and most disease states (just not right before a workout, game, or race).

That said, the NHANES 2009-2010 survey found that the average dietary fiber intake in the United States is only 16 grams per day, not even close to the recommended amount of 20 to 35 grams per day for blood sugar control and improved overall health (Hoy and Goldman 2014). Again, a great way to reach this fiber intake goal is to ensure you are consuming adequate fruits, veggies, whole grains, legumes, nuts, and seeds daily.

Spotlight on Keith LaScalea, MD

Keith LaScalea, MD, is an internist at Weill Cornell Medical College in New York City. In addition to seeing patients, Dr. LaScalea teaches and mentors medical students at the same institution. Keith is also a seasoned marathoner, who, as of January 2020, successfully completed a marathon in all 50 states. He understands the unique physical and medical needs of Masters athletes as we age.

© Keith LaScalea

What nutrition advice do you give your patients?

One thing I tell most of my patients is to eat a more plant-based diet. I am continually impressed with the science on how plant-based diets lead to health benefits. It is also easier to follow than most realize. As my patients shift to a more plant-based diet, their parameters of health, including cholesterol levels and blood sugar control, improve, and they tend to have an easier time with weight control. Many of my New York City patients also drink a fair amount of alcohol, which they often don't take into account. This is often a difficult habit to change, but if they can, it's a good place to make major improvements. The interplay between alcohol, sleep patterns, overall food intake, and fitness is something I find most people don't fully appreciate.

How do you help motivate your patients to make positive health changes?

The way I see it, if I want my patients to do something, then I also need to make and follow that same change. Then, how do I help them do it? Baby steps, then I refer them to a nutritionist for more in-depth nutrition advice. On the exercise front, we know clinically that people will stick with what they enjoy, so my advice is find something fun, make sure it is convenient, and partner with someone else for accountability.

What nutritional changes have you personally made as a Masters athlete?

I am definitely more conscious of taking in enough protein because I know adequate protein is important for muscle turnover, and considering that I eat mostly plants, I need to make sure I eat enough. I am also better about listening to my body and understanding what it needs.

The NHANES 2013-2016 results found that higher overall sodium intake increases risk of both HTN and CVD. Seventy percent of all sodium consumed is added in foods made outside the home, while only 13 to 16 percent of sodium consumed is inherently in the foods we eat, 4 to 9 percent is added in the home during food preparation, and 3 to 8 percent is added by individuals at the table (Benjamin et al. 2019). AHA states that about 77.9 million adults (1 out of 3 American adults) have high blood pressure; 47.5 percent do not have it well controlled, and an increase in incidence of HTN by 7.2% is projected by 2030.

Maintaining optimal blood pressure or lowering elevated blood pressure to reduce risk of HTN and CVD is simpler than many think. According to the guide to decreasing blood pressure distributed by the U.S. Department of Health and Human Services, we should eat more fruits, vegetables, low-fat dairy, skinless poultry and fish, nuts, legumes, and nontropical vegetable oils, and decrease our intake of saturated and trans fats, sodium, red meat, and sugar-sweetened beverages. The DASH (Dietary Approach to Stopping Hypertension) eating plan has demonstrated great success in reducing risk of CVD and similarly encourages everyone to eat four or five servings each of fruits and vegetables each day; seven or eight servings of whole grains daily; nuts, seeds, and dry beans four or five times a week; and lean meats and fish no more than twice a day. Table 3.1 shows the full DASH dietary guidelines.

TABLE 3.1   DASH Dietary Guidelines

Food group	Number of servings	Serving size
Vegetables	4 or 5 per day	1 cup raw leafy vegetable 1/2 cup cooked vegetable 6 oz (170 mL) vegetable juice
Fruits	4 or 5 per day	1 medium fruit 1/4 cup dried fruit 1/2 cup frozen or canned fruit 6 oz (170 mL) fruit juice
Nuts, seeds, and dry beans	4 or 5 per week	1/3 cup (1.5 oz) nuts 1 tbsp (1/2 oz) seeds 1/2 cup cooked beans
Grains and grain products	7 or 8 per day	1/2 cup cooked rice, pasta, cereal 1 slice of bread
Low-fat or fat-free dairy	2 or 3 per day	8 oz (240 mL) low-fat milk 1 cup low-fat yogurt 1.5 oz (45 g) low-fat cheese
Lean meats, poultry, and fish	2 per day or fewer	3 oz (90 g) cooked lean meat, skinless poultry, or fish
Fats and oils	2 or 3 per day	1 tsp soft margarine 1 tbsp low-fat mayonnaise 2 tbsp light salad dressing 1 tsp vegetable oil
Sweets	5 per week	1 tbsp sugar 1 tbsp jelly or jam 1/2 oz (15 g) sugary candy 8 oz (240 mL) lemonade

Data from National Heart, Lung, and Blood Institute; National Institutes of Health; U.S. Department of Health and Human Services.

In addition, AHA recommends maintaining a healthy weight, following a balanced and healthy eating plan, drinking alcohol only in moderation, and taking measures to decrease stress. If overweight, AHA recommends losing weight slowly, at 1/2 to 1 pound per week (and I'd say ideally in the off-season for athletes) and suggests the DASH style of eating.

The NHANES results also show that obesity is associated with higher risk of several major health issues including diabetes, HTN, hypercholesterolemia, CVD, stroke, and certain cancers, and that the prevalence of obesity is higher among adults ages 40 to 59 (42.8%) versus adults ages 20 to 39 (35.7%). For reference, obesity is defined as a body mass index (BMI) of greater than 30. BMI can be calculated as weight in kilograms divided by height in meters squared.

Spotlight on Tony Claudino

Tony Claudino is a soccer player turned triathlete and one of the founders of the Brooklyn Triathlon Club in New York City in 2004. He has been active all his life and gives back to sport. Like so many athletes I see in my practice, he also is an athlete who has had to learn to eat not only for sport performance but also for medical and health management.

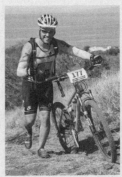

Courtesy of XTERRA.

What has your athletic journey entailed?

I've been a soccer player all my life. I played youth soccer nationally, in Olympic development, and then for four years as an NCAA athlete. Now, 25 year later, I am the oldest player on my team. As I have gotten older, I have also found marathons and triathlons. I completed my first Ironman Triathlon (one-day event consisting of a 2.4-mile swim, 112-mile bike ride, and 26.2-mile run) in Austria in 2006 and completed in Kona, Hawaii, at the Ironman World Championships in 2008.

How has your eating changed as a Masters athlete?

In my early 30s, my doctor informed me that my cholesterol levels were very high. I am forever grateful to him for recommending that I meet with a dietitian. I really wanted to try to lower my cholesterol nutritionally, and working with you as my dietitian has had a major positive impact on my life. I am Portuguese and my wife is Czech, so we had been eating a good deal of meat, but I reduced that gradually and have been pescatarian for six or seven years. Each time we met, you helped me make a few changes: more whole grains, less red meat, more beans and oats, and more good fats. These changes always felt doable, and I looked at them the way I do training progressions. I have been impressed by how making nutritional changes has drastically lowered my cholesterol and has also helped me perform my best athletically. I recover better and have more energy now than I did 10 to 15 years ago.

each of whom have been active for their entire lives and are an inspiration to athletes everywhere.

As Norman Goluskin states beautifully in his sidebar on the next page, eating healthfully is important to our overall health, athletic performance, and longevity in sport, but moderation is just as important. Allowing ourselves to eat and enjoy the foods that we want and not obsess about every morsel we put into our mouths is just as important to our overall health. We will hear many athletes discuss their relationship to food, including their struggles with eating disorders, throughout this book, and specifically in chapter 10.

The "Ideal" Diet

Over the past several years, much research has been done on finding the "ideal" diet and macronutrient ratios for weight loss and weight maintenance. Let's address the important findings.

The National Weight Control Registry tracks individuals who have successfully lost an average of 66 pounds and kept it off for an average of 5.5 years. It looks for patterns in success in order to help shape recommendations for others seeking long-term weight loss success. The average age of these members is 45 years for women and 49 years for men. Here are the major findings from the registry.

- Ninety-eight percent of individuals report having modified their food intake.
- Ninety-four percent increased their overall amount of exercise to achieve weight loss.
- Ninety percent report exercising for about one hour per day, mainly by walking.
- Seventy-eight percent eat breakfast every day.
- Seventy-five percent check their weight once per week.

Another large study looked at eating patterns and the effect of different proportions of carbohydrate, protein, and fat on long-term weight loss and weight maintenance in individuals from eight European countries (Larsen et al. 2010). They induced an 8 percent weight loss in overweight individuals over a 26-week study, then randomly assigned individuals to one of five maintenance diet conditions: low protein, low glycemic index (GI); low protein, high GI; higher protein, low GI; higher protein, high GI; and a control group. These researchers found a modest improvement in weight maintenance in individuals when they were assigned a moderately increased protein and modest GI diet.

One year earlier, Sacks et al. (2009) reported their findings on the effects of different percentages of carbohydrate, protein, and fat intake on long-term weight and laboratory results. They enrolled 800 overweight and obese individuals between the ages of 30 and 70 and asked them to follow one of several weight loss diets (table 4.1). During the study, they conducted individual sessions for each weight loss participant every eight weeks for two years, and offered group counseling sessions weekly for six months and then every other week for the reminder of the two-year study duration. All dietary conditions followed the guidelines and included less than

Spotlight on Norman Goluskin

Norman Goluskin became an athlete and advocate of exercise for all in his 30s, sat on the board of directors for the New York Road Runners (NYRR) for 20 years, and has been a board member of the Mohonk Preserve since 1999. Athletically, Norman ran in the first five-borough NYC Marathon in 1976, has a marathon personal record of 2:41 (Boston), has set age-group world records as part of 4 × 800 meter relays in his 60s and 70s, and most recently won gold medals for age 80 and up at the National Championships in both the 5,000 and 10,000 meter and silver in the 1,500 meter. He was integral in the formation of the NYRR Children's Running Program and the fundraising arm, Team for Kids, which now serves 250,000 children nationwide. Norman was very serious when he said that his goal was to get every single kid in the world to be active. His humble and inclusive view of runners and all humans is both refreshing and invigorating.

Norman shared his secrets for long-term athletic success.

1. Just show up.
2. If you can't get faster, get older!

What was your progression as an athlete?

As a kid, I literally ran to the store when my mom asked me to go to buy milk, but when I made the track team my calves started to hurt, so that didn't stick. Thereafter I made the swim team but didn't stick with that either. When I was 37 years old, I was in between marriages, started exercising for stress relief, and began running around the track. At first, by the end of a mile I thought I was going to die. Then I ran 1.5 miles and realized I wasn't actually going to die, but honestly thought I might hurt for the rest of my life. Then one week I joined a friend for a 5-mile run and somehow loved it! The rest, as they say, is history.

What do you see as the positive aspects of being a Masters athlete?

I ran in the 10k road championships in April 2019, and our ages were written on our backs. Younger people ran by cheering, saying I was an inspiration. I have never thought of myself as an inspiration, but I suppose people think it is impressive that at 80 I can still stand upright and keep running. I was always a good runner but not a great runner, and now is my chance to be highly competitive.

TABLE 4.1 Macronutrient Ratios for Different Diets

Dietary condition	Fat intake (%)	Protein intake (%)	Carbohydrate intake (%)
Low fat, low protein	20	15	65
Low fat, high protein	20	25	55
High fat, average protein	40	15	45
High fat, high protein	40	25	35

Has your nutrition helped you over your lifetime and athletic career?

I have never been a big fan of veggies, which I recognize is unfortunate, but I do make a concerted effort to eat them. For years I thought pizza was a food group. Fortunately, I am married to a woman who has more interest in proper diet, so I have eaten better over the years because of her. Kidding aside, I eat reasonably healthfully. Toast and a banana before my morning run, then for my postrun breakfast I eat oatmeal with berries and coffee. Lunch is more varied: maybe a tuna sandwich, sometimes salmon. For dinner, I will eat fish or some type of protein and rice or other carbohydrate. My wife will make string beans and will tell me I should eat more of them, and so I will have some.

How have you altered your nutritional intake as a Masters athlete?

My father died at 53 from heart disease, so I was aware of my family risk of heart disease from an early age. In my 70s, a cardiologist told me my calcium score was really high and to follow the Mediterranean diet. The way I am wired, if it is worth doing it is worth overdoing, so I immediately went to eating only "properly." Pretty soon thereafter I woke up to the fact that I didn't have to eat perfectly; I just needed more balance. It was better not to be at either extreme. I am still running competitively at 80 and feeling pretty good, so I guess I ended up OK.

What motivates you to keep running?

To this day, all of my best friends have come out of the running community. We are a diverse group who seem to have good core values. In running, it doesn't matter what you do for a living, who is richer, who is older, or where you came from; it is all about who you can run with. We all care about health, respect for other people, and respect for nature and the outdoors, and that is what matters most.

Norman's Favorite Postrace Meal

My running partners* clearly have their favorite greasy breakfast after a race, but I don't. I think other people have incorporated the thought that food is part of the reward for running, but I am a one-dimensional guy.

*I run because I love it,
And food is food and is separate from when or why I run,
Just like running shoes are running shoes.*

* Roger Robinson, who you will meet in chapter 11, is one of Norman's running partners as well as his running coach and postrace breakfast companion.

8 percent saturated fat, more than 20 grams total fiber, and less than 150 mg cholesterol. By six months, the average weight loss across all diets was 13 pounds (6 kg, or 7 percent of initial body weight). By about 12 months, weight regain began for many individuals. By two years, the overall weight loss remained equal at 9 pounds (4 kg) net loss for all, and satiety, hunger, and satisfaction were equal for all diets.

They did not find any effect of higher versus lower protein, higher versus lower fat, or percentage of food from carbohydrate on weight loss or waist circumference. After the two-year study period, all groups lowered their fasting insulin, triglycerides, and blood pressure, while the lower fat diets led to the greatest decrease in LDL (the bad cholesterol) and the lowest carbohydrate diet led to the greatest increase in HDL (the good cholesterol). All diets led to weight loss and improved lipids, and the biggest takeaway is that the greatest results were seen in those who attended the most group counseling sessions, regardless of which dietary condition they had been assigned to.

The conclusion Sacks et al. (2009, p. 871) made from this is that any diet undertaken "with enthusiasm and persistence, can be effective." They also noted individual differences and preferences between dietary eating patterns, and recognized that each person's personal food preferences and inclinations should be taken into account in order to increase their chances of long-term success. That is not to say that the macronutrient composition of Masters athletes' diets has no importance—it clearly does; but so does choosing an eating style that resonates with you and fits your preferences

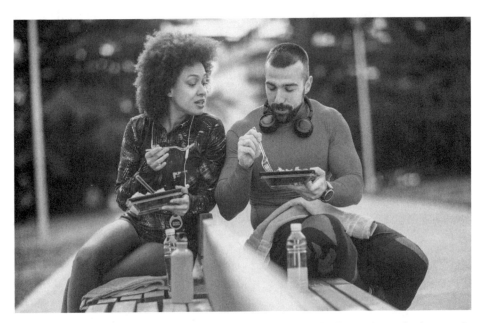

Choosing foods based on your preferences and needs is the best way to fuel properly and consistently.
EXTREME-PHOTOGRAPHER/iStock/Getty Images

and lifestyle. The next three chapters will explain macronutrient intake and timing including our increasing protein needs as we age, and the importance of spreading our protein intake throughout our day.

It is important to keep in mind that there is no one diet or macronutrient eating pattern that is the only or the best diet for all athletes or for humans as a whole. Successful dieters and individuals with lower overall risk of disease, however, have in common some overriding nutrition principles, which have led to the following overall health recommendations for a Healthy Eating Plate (Harvard School of Public Health 2011; figure 4.1):

- Fill half your plate with fruits and vegetables (and eat them).
- Eat a wide variety in color and type of produce.
- Fill a quarter of your plate with whole grains.
- Fill a quarter of your plate with protein (fish, poultry, beans, nuts).
- Avoid or limit red meat and processed meat.
- Use healthy, plant-based oils such as olive, canola, sunflower, and peanut oil in moderation.
- Decrease intake of hydrogenated and trans fats.
- Drink water, coffee, and tea.
- Limit sugar-sweetened drinks.

Healthy Eating Plate

Use healthy oils (like olive and canola oil) for cooking, on salad, and at the table. Limit butter. Avoid trans fat.

The more veggies – and the greater the variety – the better. Potatoes and French fries don't count.

Eat plenty of fruits of all colors.

STAY ACTIVE!

Drink water, tea, or coffee (with little or no sugar). Limit milk/dairy (1-2 servings/day) and juice (1 small glass/day). Avoid sugary drinks.

Eat a variety of whole grains (like whole-wheat bread, whole-grain pasta, and brown rice). Limit refined grains (like white rice and white bread).

Choose fish, poultry, beans, and nuts; limit red meat and cheese; avoid bacon, cold cuts, and other processed meats.

FIGURE 4.1 Healthy Eating Plate.

This is to be used only as a starting point because athletes' daily and meal-by-meal nutritional needs vary based on many factors including height, weight, age, gender, and activity level. As we will discuss in detail in chapter 5, many athletes will need to increase their proportion of carbs and possibly decrease their portion of veggies in order to meet their needs during times of heavy training.

Spotlight on Meb Keflezighi

Meb Keflezighi is the only runner ever to win both the Boston and New York City marathons and also medal in the Olympic marathon. In addition to his running accomplishments, Meb has written two books, *Meb for Mortals* and *26 Marathons*. Most importantly, Meb is a caring, honest, and genuine husband, father, and man, with whom I thoroughly enjoyed speaking.

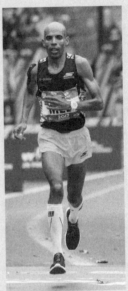

As we began, and before I was even able to thank him for agreeing to speak with me, Meb led with this: "We have a lot in common! We are both the same age, and we are both athletes who fell in love with running in seventh grade. We have both run the Boston and NYC marathons. The only difference is that I have made the Olympics. Otherwise we have been on the same journey." After a good laugh on my part, we began.

How do you think about running a marathon?

A marathon is a marathon one way or the other—it is 26.2 miles—and there is no shortcut for that. We all go through   Elsa/Getty Images
struggles and challenges while training for and during the marathon itself. No matter whether you are in the lead, the middle of the pack, or the back of the pack, that part of the experience is the same. Running a marathon will teach you a lot about yourself.

What is your nutritional intake on a day-to-day basis?

My wife is responsible for all of our daily meals. She does a great job of balancing cooking for the kids and for herself and me, and keeping us all eating healthy. I am fortunate that growing up, my mom cooked all of our food from scratch. I have 10 brothers and sisters, and we always had a delicious homemade dish Mom had made for us. We had pasta with fresh homemade sauce, a lot of chicken, greens, salads, and potatoes. We did not grow up eating anything heated from frozen, and we don't feed that to our family now. If you grow up eating fried, processed, and frozen foods, you will not know any better, and that is too bad.

How has your eating changed as a Masters athlete?

I know from years of training and racing that nutrition is important and becomes even more important as we age. I have a sweet tooth, but we keep a bowl of fruit strate and is critical for high-intensity exercise performance and recovery. The report goes on to say that failure to consume adequate carbohydrate between sessions leads only to suboptimally replenished glycogen (energy) stores, greater fatigue, and worsened performance in subsequent sessions, especially when exercise is performed regularly—that is, when there is little time to recover from one session before tackling another. In chapter 13 we will explore recovery as the holy grail of longevity in sport, but first let's hear from an amazing athlete who speaks of her evolving relationship with and increasing intake of carbs as a Masters athlete.

History and Evolution of Carbohydrate Loading

As we discuss the importance of available carbohydrate to athletic performance, a logical question becomes, *How can we get our bodies to store more of this precious fuel source?* This question was first studied and written about in the late 1960s as scientists noted that while an untrained individual typically stores 80 to 90 millimole per kilogram of muscle glycogen, trained athletes increased that ability to 125 millimole per kilogram. This is a huge storage improvement and provided athletes enough glycogen to get through 60 to 90 minutes of moderate-intensity exercise. For events lasting longer than 90 minutes, athletes reported increased fatigue and decreased work capacity likely due to decreased muscle glycogen availability. It was found that after only a three- to five-day period of increased carbohydrate intake (at 8 g/kg body weight/day) accompanied by reduced training volume, muscle glycogen stores increased even further to greater than 200 millimole per kilogram. This was great information in the world of performance nutrition and exercise performance, and many athletes (including Polly de Mille, who we heard from in chapter 2) describe following this carbohydrate-loading protocol to a T for many years. However, as any of you who have ever tried this can attest, the protocol is not easy to follow and in fact is prohibitive to effective training for anyone who competes often. Additionally, since every 1 gram of glycogen is stored with 2 to 3 grams of water, this carbohydrate loading leads to a 1 to 2 percent increase in body weight over the few days that is it being done just prior to an important competition (Bartlett, Hawley, and Morton 2015). If this topic interests you, state tuned; we will cover the evolution of carbohydrate loading in more detail in chapter 11.

Choosing Your Carbohydrate Fuel

The necessity of carbohydrate for optimal fueling and for improving overall performance has been well documented since the 1930s. A pretraining carbohydrate meal increases muscle glycogen blunt fatty acid mobilization, which is a good thing because carbs transfer energy faster than fats. Many athletes find they need (and then want) to eat three meals and two or three

Spotlight on Sarah True

Sarah True represented the United States in Olympic triathlon competition in both 2012 and 2016. She placed fourth at the Ironman World Championships in Kona, Hawaii, in 2018, which was her Ironman debut. Sarah candidly shares her early nutritional struggles and speaks of eventually coming to peace with eating what her body needs, which includes much more carbohydrate than she was initially taught, and fueling for both life and elite competition.

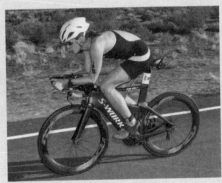

Donald Miralle/Getty Images

How have your overall nutrition and daily fueling changed since you became a Masters athlete?

My biggest nutrition shift is that as a younger athlete, I was concerned I would end up carrying more weight if I ate more carbohydrate, and ironically, I have found that I recover faster, my training quality is higher, I am more consistent, and it is easier for me to maintain a stable weight when I allow myself to eat the carbs I need. My carbohydrate intake goes up as my training increases, and it decreases during the off-season, but I don't track numbers or grams; at this point it is pretty intuitive, which is how it should be! The idea that we "should" be feeling shameful about food and eating is disturbing. I don't think of foods as being good or bad anymore, and that has changed my relationship with food and made eating much less stressful. Of course, I think of some foods as more nutritious and others as less nutritious, but I don't believe in cheat days, and I don't believe in depriving yourself of anything you love. There is a lot of baggage in sports around body weight and appearance and body dysmorphia, and we need to change that! My second big sport nutrition shift was becoming aware of and staying on top of getting in enough calories and carbohydrate during intense training and racing.

How did you break free from the carb phobia and underfueling messaging?

The beauty of being a woman with years of athletic experience is that I have let go of allowing social and external cues to guide my fueling habits. This is not easy to do, because we are all inundated with messages about nutrition. In the past, I tried to follow a restrictive diet per my coaches' recommendation, only to find myself with cravings, frequent sinus infections, and feeling terrible during training. My weight also fluctuated a lot, and I would put on weight in the off-season. When I suffered a broken hip after a minor bike crash going 10 miles per hour, it finally registered for me. I abandoned this "diet" mentality, went back to intuitive eating, healed my injury, and my training improved pretty quickly. I have learned how to fuel myself, both as a person and as a high-performance athlete.

What would you say to other athletes struggling to figure out their best nutritional intake?

This has become part of my mission, because it is amazing how athletes (or people in general) overvalue anecdotal reports from other elite athletes or coaches, even ferred fuel source by the body, in part likely because carbohydrate requires less energy per unit of oxygen. For athletes who know they are going to need to perform under conditions of low carbohydrate availability (such as in a multiple-day stage race), practicing this nutritional strategy may offer some metabolic benefit when limited carbohydrate is available. For the rest of us, although increasing fat oxidation may sound appealing, total energy expenditure is not significantly different and RPE is increased on a higher-fat versus a higher-carbohydrate diet, which is likely to lead to an unintentional decrease in training volume, intensity, or both.

In terms of fully reviewing the efficacy of higher-fat versus traditional higher-carb diets for athletes, despite the hopes and research, there is little evidence at this time to advocate the use of a high-fat, low-carb nutritional strategy for performance enhancement, although more research is needed in terms of any potential benefit for moderate-intensity, ultradistance events, which use a higher percentage of fat as fuel to begin with.

Food and Mood: Carbohydrate Is Not Just for Muscles

As Sarah True highlighted so beautifully in speaking about her own life, another important area of interest is decreased mood accompanying a low carbohydrate diet or a state of low carbohydrate availability. Achten and colleagues (2004) studied runners on both high carbohydrate (8.5 g/kg/day) and low-carbohydrate (5.4 g/kg/day) diets and found clear evidence of both better physical performance and improved mood state on the higher carbohydrate diet despite matched total energy intakes on both (i.e., higher fat, higher protein intake to make up for lower carb intake). In addition to improved global mood with adequate total carbohydrate intake, these studies found decreased incidence and reports of fatigue (lower RPE) in athletes, both during exercise and at rest on higher carb diets. They noted that others have studied this and found similar results in swimmers, rowers, cyclists, and runners. Such studies support the idea that training in a low carbohydrate state may play an important role in the development of overreaching in athletes. Knowing this, it is paramount that athletes and those working with them ensure adequate total carbohydrate intake daily in order to reduce risk of overreaching as well as to maintain adequate mood state and performance during training sessions.

In my professional experience, athletes are often surprised when I calculate their individual needs and inform them of their total carbohydrate goals. Because of false notions involving carbohydrate and weight and because of other current societal messaging on carbohydrate, many athletes follow plans that result in molecular level changes but not overall performance advantages, and they are chronically running on less-than-ideal fueling. Especially for Masters athletes, this becomes a long-term health, mood, and performance issue. Thankfully, it is one you can reverse with greater understanding of your needs and a quick bit of math in order to calculate them.

After reviewing all available science and noting practical evidence in working with professional, elite, and recreational athletes for more than 15 years, the question I ask is, "Will any particular nutrition intervention enhance your

Spotlight on Gordon Bakoulis

Gordon Bakoulis is a five-time U.S. Olympic marathon trials qualifier, running coach, editorial director for the New York Road Runners (NYRR), and a self-proclaimed carbohydrate lover. Gordon also ran in the 10,000 meter Olympic trials in 1992 and was first in her group at the New York City Marathon at 40 years old, when she ran an amazing 2:41.43. She is also the author of the books *Cross-Training* and *How to Train For and Run Your Best Marathon*, and she is an example of

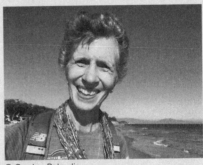
© Gordon Bakoulis

someone who embodies the true essence of love of sport and a refreshing no-nonsense attitude about health and nutrition.

How have your eating habits changed throughout your lifetime?

I was born in 1961, and nutrition just wasn't being spoken about the same way it is now. I grew up eating TV dinners; that was normal. Everyone's lunches were sandwiches on white bread with Yodels or Ring Dings. I was raised that you have to try everything, but fortunately, I was not forced to finish my plate, and we never forced our kids to finish theirs either. In college, I had an eating disorder for just over a year. For me, it was about control and being the best at something. I decided that if I couldn't be the smartest or fastest, I could be the thinnest. What pulled me out of the eating disorder was actually my running, because after a while I just couldn't run anymore. I enjoyed running for stress relief and also wanted to be competitive, so I began to eat more. Running became my motivation to get better. I knew what it felt like not to eat all day and then go for a run, and I knew I didn't want to do that anymore.

Tell me about your daily nutrition habits now, as a Masters runner.

I always ate a carb-heavy diet and still do. I would say that I have a good runner's diet. I have a meat-centric dinner three times a week, and the other nights are more plant-based. I try to include deep greens and kale, plus orange and yellow vegetables such as sweet potatoes daily, and I make sure I include protein: meat or tofu and nuts. At this point in my life, I feel mindful and knowledgeable about my nutrition. At the end of the day, I am checking off the boxes on my fruits and vegetables; I am thinking, "Have I had enough today?" I also have dessert pretty much every day—usually a bowl of ice cream.

7 | Healthy Fat

The topic of dietary fat intake has felt like a bit of a roller-coaster ride over the past three decades. In the 1980s dietary fat was shunned, because higher total energy intake as well as diets with higher animal fat and saturated fat were linked to higher rates of heart disease and other chronic diseases; fat-free foods became ubiquitous. The unintended consequence of this was a movement toward diets with higher refined carbohydrate and foods with their natural (and even healthy) fat replaced with refined carbohydrate and sugar (Liu et al. 2017). Throughout this relatively short lived fat-free craze, it seemed that most people were not focusing on the quality of their food, rather only the number of grams of fat each food contained. This led to higher intakes of processed foods and refined sugar, which we now know leads to dyslipidemia (lower healthy HDL and higher triglycerides), and resulted in poor health and performance. A great majority of the U.S. population learned to avoid foods that are healthy but calorically dense, including nuts, seeds, avocados, and olive and vegetable oils, which only drove U.S. obesity rates and energy intake higher than ever (Liu et al. 2017).

Next, we moved into a high-fat food craze with the likes of the Atkins diet and ketogenic-type diets, which caused many to greatly increase their fat intake from all sources and to shun healthy foods including all fruits and most veggies and grains. This shifted the conversation toward the benefits of eating adequate dietary fat every day and the different effects fat intake has on our health based on dietary source (enter labeling of fat sources as "good" and "bad" fats).

That said, some athletes still doubt the necessity of dietary fat, and some are reluctant to give up their high-fat eating patterns. Before we delve into the science behind fat, we turn now to an amazing athlete and advocate of clean and fair sport for all, Kara Goucher, to hear about her transition from following the low-fat diet once considered healthy to embracing a higher fat diet and reaping the benefits thereof.

Spotlight on Kara Goucher

Kara Goucher is a two-time Olympian and world champion. She represented the United States at the 2008 Beijing Summer Olympics in both the 10,000 meter and 5,000 meter, and at the 2012 Olympics in London in the marathon. Kara made her marathon debut in 2008, when she came in an astounding third in the New York City Marathon, then went on to finish third at the Boston Marathon in 2009. Kara gave birth to her son, Colton (Colt), in September 2010, then came back to set a personal record at the Boston Marathon in 2011. Kara is also an advocate of clean sport and a cohost of the Clean Sport Collective podcast (@cleansportco). We had an honest conversation about her running, fueling, and coming back after having her baby.

Christian Petersen/Getty Images

How has your nutritional intake changed to support your needs as a Masters runner?

I have been running for a really long time, and my nutrition has always been pretty good overall. That said, as a professional athlete and marathoner I had to learn the importance of eating more protein and more fat, and then of paying attention to my recovery nutrition. Mostly, I have learned that all of the things that when I was younger I could get away with—say, a little less sleep, not fueling well, or forgetting my water bottle on an 18-mile run—I can no longer get away with and have therefore stopped doing. As I am getting older, I find that I really need to pay more attention to meeting my nutrition and hydration needs. I don't go running on an empty stomach anymore because if I do, I feel lightheaded. If I don't fuel well during a long run, I'll bonk before 16 miles and feel like crap for three days. I also need to consume calories and protein within an hour after all of my workouts. All of it seems to have a greater impact on my recovery and training now. When I was training for the 2016 Olympic Trials at age 37, I was training as hard as ever but was really diligent about taking fuel during workouts and staying on top of my recovery nutrition, plus using compression socks and napping. Basically, I was taking really good care of my body, and it paid off.

Have you shifted your overall intake of any one macronutrient as a Masters athlete?

My first professional coach had us speak to a registered dietitian, who said we needed to be eating avocado and nuts and other sources of fat. At first it kind of blew my mind, because when I was younger, I went through the whole phase of thinking fat was bad. There was a boom of non-fat foods and "fat is bad" thinking, and we all fell for it. Eventually, I started reading more about it, and other athletes eating those foods assured me that I would feel better and be leaner, so by 2007 to 2008 I tried it, and my performance got better. It was so much better overall to eat yogurt that tastes good and to put avocado on my sandwich. Everything tasted so much better. Then, as I got older, I realized that as I started eating more fat my joints feel better, my skin is better, my recovery definitely is better, and I feel better overall. I eat pretty much everything now. I don't avoid anything. At 40, I wanted to run the Olympic Trials in the marathon again—just to know I could do it—and again went to a registered dietitian. I had thought I was getting enough protein because I was eating it every night at dinner, but she said I needed more, and especially since I was getting older, I needed to make sure I ate protein throughout my day. She asked me to shoot for 20 grams of protein at breakfast, then another 30 at lunch and dinner. At first it was shocking to me to see how far off I was, but she gave me lists of foods that have the amount of protein I need at any given meal, and that was helpful. Otherwise, I would have just started eating a lot of chicken.

How has your in-race fueling strategy changed over the years?

When I first started marathoning, I used water and gels, because sport drinks taste like a melted popsicle to me and I just couldn't take in enough, which meant I wasn't taking enough fluid or calories. That wasn't good. Then I found Nuun Endurance, which has a lighter flavor. I used it for my race in Houston, and it worked well. When I first started marathoning, I used to take a swig or two from my bottle and then just chuck it, but I quickly realized I needed to get in more and more calories. Now, since I recently started training for ultras, I did my first three-hour training run, and have a new respect for the four- to five-hour marathoners, because you really have to plan and fuel for them. Also, you are alone in your head for so long, and I now know how hard that is.

Have you experienced any nutrition-related race-day disasters?

I recently ran a trail marathon at altitude and underestimated my needs. I went through my gels and liquids like crazy. At [my road marathon] 5:30 pace, I was trying not to break stride. Now that I am training for longer trail races and am running a lot slower, I need to practice taking in solid foods.

Tell me about your return to running a marathon PR after having your baby.

I don't recommend that anyone else do what I did here. I was under pressure with my job as a professional runner and with my contract with my sponsor, Nike. I had a 6.5-month-old, I was running 120 miles per week, and I ran 2:24. You may say that sounds impressive, and I guess it does, but long term it was not a good choice. I recommend that others learn from my experience and not be in a rush. New-mom runners should be patient and take their time to enjoy their baby and not add more stress to that time. My hope is that sponsors learn from this as well and stop putting pressure on female athletes to return to top performance so quickly after having a baby. Because I was under pressure to return to running and competing quickly, I got a stress fracture in my femur by the time Colt was 10 months old. It then became a chronic weakness in my hip that I have been dealing with since. It was physically not good for my body long term, and it was also not good for me mentally to be under such stress to run. Running 120 miles per week and trying to be a new mom was not easy, and because of it I was not able to enjoy what was happening in my life. Again, it may sound impressive, but I can't stress enough that I do not recommend it to anyone.

Kara's Favorite Postrace Meal

My favorite thing after a race is to get loaded nachos and eat it as my dinner. Definitely not stadium nachos with bad cheese—good-quality nachos with beans, chicken, and guacamole.

With Kara's personal nutrition journey and purposeful increase in dietary fat intake as a starting point, I clarify in this chapter why athletes in both extreme camps are better off moderating their fat intake. I also hope that as athletes continue to look at the science, they will listen to the health organizations' practical and moderate recommended range of dietary fat intake of 20 to 35 percent of total daily food, with a focus on polyunsaturated fats.

Benefits of Dietary Fats

As always, our goals as Masters athletes include maintaining an adequate diet both in terms of total energy availability (calories) as well as in all macro- and micronutrients. As such, dietary fat is an "important and necessary component of a healthy diet" (Thomas, Erdman, and Burke 2016). Dietary fat not only provides us with essential energy, but also allows us to absorb fat-soluble vitamins, is integral in hormone production, provides us with essential nutrients that we require in order to continue to make cell membranes, and last, but certainly not least, provides us with delicious tastes and satiety after eating. Before we discuss the specific dietary needs of Masters athletes for fat, we'll review the types of fat we eat and overall healthy guidelines for fat intake.

Understanding Dietary Fat

The Academy of Nutrition and Dietetics (AND) recommends including 15 to 20 percent of our daily calories from monounsaturated fatty acids (MUFA), including nuts, avocado, and peanut butter, due to their ability to help us increase our HDL (good cholesterol) and reduce risk of heart disease, while limiting our intake of saturated fat to less than 10 percent of total calories or nutritional intake per day, and trans fat to less than 1 percent of total calories or intake for the day (Gordon 2019). The AND also encourages increased consumption of omega-3 polyunsaturated fat and omega-3 fat from fatty fish, walnuts, flaxseed, chia seeds, hemp seeds, and eggs, due to many health benefits, including reducing cholesterol levels and lowering the risk of heart disease and inflammation in the body.

All fats have a combination of polyunsaturated, monounsaturated, and saturated fatty acids, albeit in different amounts. The Dietary Guidelines for Americans recommend about 5 tablespoons of fats per day, which equals about 600 calories' worth or about 30 percent of dietary intake for a person with a typical daily need for 2,000 calories (Goldman 2016). They also recommend limiting saturated fat intake to less than 10 percent of total calories. Essential fatty acids, including linoleic acid and alpha-linolenic acid, and polyunsaturated fats, such as corn, sunflower, and soybean oils, are recommended over other sources of fat, as is consuming fatty fish twice a week. Other health-promoting fat sources to include are flaxseeds and walnuts; olive, canola, peanut, sunflower, and safflower oils; as well as and avocados and peanut butter. Most athletes should choose 1 to 2 servings of these healthy fats with most meals and snacks. Overall, they recommend a plant-based diet and a reduction in animal fat intake.

All types of dietary fat provide 9 calories of energy per gram, but that is where the similarities between types of fat end. Poly- and monounsaturated fat include those that are typically liquid at room temperature but solid when refrigerated or chilled. These are often referred to as healthy fats, and they include the omega-3 and omega-6 fatty acids that have been shown to reduce the amount of LDL (bad cholesterol) in our bodies, thus lowering our risk of heart disease, stroke, and diabetes (American Heart Association 2017). These important fats also provide us with much-needed vitamin E and help us absorb fat-soluble vitamins, including vitamins A, D, E, and K. Foods that contain polyunsaturated fat include soybeans or edamame; corn; sunflower, olive, canola, peanut, and sesame oils; walnuts, flax, sunflower, and other nuts and seeds; and tofu. Foods rich in monounsaturated fat include olive, canola, peanut, safflower, and sesame oils (American Heart Association 2017).

The American Heart Association also recommends limiting saturated fat to 5 to 6 percent of total caloric intake per day and eliminating trans fat as much as possible, ideally down to zero, due to their undesirable ability to increase LDL and decrease HDL, which then increases our risk of heart disease, stroke, and type 2 diabetes. Saturated fat is called such because its molecules are saturated with hydrogen atoms. Foods high in saturated fat include animal meats, butter, cheese, lard, cream, fried foods, and coconut and palm oils. Some tropical oils that are high in saturated fat, including palm, palm kernel, and coconut, can trigger the liver to produce more cholesterol. Trans fat is no longer classified as generally recognized as safe (GRAS) in our food supply according

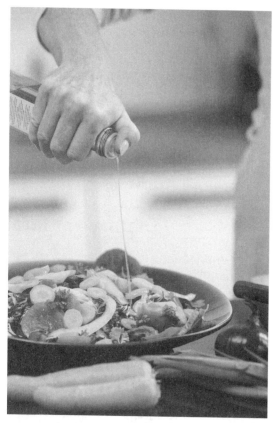

Olive oil is a good source of both polyunsaturated and monounsaturated fat.
Plattform/Getty Images

TABLE 7.1   Dietary Fat Sources by Type

EAT MORE		EAT LESS	
Foods high in mono-unsaturated fat	**Foods high in poly-unsaturated fat**	**Foods high in satu-rated fat**	**Foods high in trans fat**

Nuts
Olive oil
Canola oil
Olives
Avocados
Peanut butter
Safflower oil
Sunflower oil
	Fatty fish (salmon,
	  mackerel, herring,
	  sardines, trout)
	Walnuts
	Flaxseeds
	Eggs fortified with
	  omega-3
	Seeds (flax, chia,
	  hemp)
	Canola oil
	Tofu
		Coconut oil
		Palm oil
		Kernel oil
		Animal meat
		Milk, whole or 2%
		Cheese
		Butter
		Cream
		Poultry skin
		Some store-bought
		  baked goods
		Fried foods
			Foods with partially
			  hydrogenated oils
			Margarine
			Store-bought baked
			  goods
			Fast food and fried
			  foods

to the U.S. Food and Drug Administration (FDA) and is now restricted or banned in many countries, states, and cities.

Trans fat is found in fried foods, margarines, and many packaged foods, including cookies, crackers, and donuts. Avoid food that has hydrogenated and partially hydrogenated oils on the food label ingredient list. It is important to review the ingredient list because food labels can legally say the product has 0 grams of trans fat per serving as long as it actually contains less than 0.5 grams.

Overall, it is advisable to replace most saturated and trans fat with poly- and monounsaturated fat to improve heart health and your lipid profile. The American Heart Association recommends consuming oils with less than 4 grams of saturated fat per tablespoon. See table 7.1 for a list of types of fat and each type's most common food.

Dietary Fat Intake Needs

Recommendations for athletes' dietary fat intake range from a minimum of 20 percent to a more typical 25 to 30 percent of total energy intake across almost all ages and sports (Thomas, Erdman, and Burke 2016). Ingesting any less than 20 percent of total calories from fat will not lead to any performance advantage but will lead to a reduction in vitamin, nutrient, and essential fatty acid intake that can be detrimental to overall health and long-term athletic performance. Only during acute periods of carbohydrate loading prior to an event or competition would a lower fat diet be advisable for athletes.

Dietary fat oxidation rates and needs will vary by athlete, sport, and training phase or block, but two facts remain true: fat continues to be a major fuel source for athletes, and adequate intake is imperative for performance and recovery to decrease inflammation and for longevity in sport.

Another specific benefit for athletes is that omega-3 fat intake has been shown to help decrease inflammation, may delay or reduce muscle soreness and stiffness, may help prevent immunosuppression often seen following prolonged or exhaustive exercise, and may help to preserve joint mobility (Thomas, Erdman, and Burke 2016).

As we have already seen, the topic of dietary fat intake as well as that of optimal body fat and body composition for athletes quickly becomes convoluted. Overall, dietary fat needs will range between 20 and 35 percent of total intake for different athletes and will depend on each athlete's overall training and calorie demands, phase of training, and body composition goals. Occasionally, dietary fat intake of more than 35 percent of total calories may be required by athletes who have higher total calorie needs, which works as long as they continue to meet their individual needs for both protein and carbohydrate and are consuming a large proportion of this fat from good sources including fatty fish, avocado, nuts, seeds, and other plant sources. However, all athletes need both adequate dietary fat intake and body fat percentage to maintain intramuscular triglycerides, meet energy demands, and maintain optimal health (Thomas, Erdman, and Burke 2016).

As discussed in chapter 5, research shows that high-fat diets do not lead to performance benefits at lower intensities, impedes high-intensity exercise performance, and reduces metabolic flexibility as carbohydrate metabolism is thereafter down-regulated (decreased) when glycogen is available (Thomas, Erdman, and Burke 2016). Furthermore, research consistently shows that a moderate- to high-carbohydrate diet (at least 5-8 g of carbohydrate/kg [2-4 g/lb] of body weight/day) is warranted in order to prevent the negative consequences of chronic, training-induced glycogen depletion (Tiller et al. 2019). Endurance athletes who remain interested in testing out this high-fat, low-carb eating strategy should first and foremost ensure they are meeting their daily calorie needs in order to facilitate recovery from prolonged and repeated training sessions.

While it is true that endurance and ultraendurance athletes are generally working at an intensity at which they burn a higher percentage of free fatty acid as fuel, they still require adequate total carbohydrate in order to meet their needs during periods of higher-intensity training and racing. (It is important to note that this has scarcely been studied in ultraendurance athletes and should be "practiced tentatively" [Tiller et al. 2019, page 14], not consistently.) Athletes interested in experimenting with completing some selected lower-intensity training sessions in a lower carbohydrate and higher fat intake state (fasted morning workouts or lower carbohydrate state for the second workout of the day) in order to enhance fat oxidation capacity should do so with specificity and with adequate refueling and rest between these sessions and higher-intensity or key workouts. The data have consistently shown that although significant metabolic adaptations are seen following a brief (five-day) period of higher dietary fat intake. Despite the fact that this increased fat oxidation persists after adequate carbohydrate is restored, there is no evidence that fat adaptation benefits cycling performance (Burke et al. 2000). That said, we know without a shadow of a doubt that training in a low carbohydrate availability state will compromise high-intensity performance and decrease an athlete's ability to maintain a high work rate, so never attempt any key or high-intensity sessions in a low carbohydrate availability state (fasted or depleted).

In addition, glycogen depletion has been shown to increase cortisol levels and lead to disturbances in the immune system, leaving athletes more likely to pick up a cold or other illness. These problems are seen most often when exercise bouts lasting more than 90 minutes are completed without adequate nutrition fuel or when this practice is repeated often (Tiller et al. 2019). In fact, during the past decade, although the available research on training low (purposefully undergoing training sessions in a state of low carbohydrate availability) has shown training adaptations including an increase in lipid oxidation rate, they always come at the price of lowering maximum training intensity (Bartlett, Hawley, and Morton 2015). And while some research has shown that implementing carbohydrate rinsing and taking additional caffeine before training low sessions can help counteract some of this decrease in performance intensity, it is unclear how much these strategies prevent increased muscle breakdown and decrease immune function when practicing frequent or prolonged low carbohydrate availability sessions. Therefore, athletes should only undertake these sessions periodically and strategically to both avoid the negative consequences and to ensure that their capacity to oxidize (use) carbohydrate is not blunted when they need it most—on race day (Bartlett, Hawley, and Morton 2015).

Many seasoned athletes may have already realized that they feel and perform their best during training sessions and races or competitions that follow a high intake of carbohydrate, rather than high intake of fat or no intake at all. The science backs that up, and that is where most of us should train and race *most* of the time.

Unfortunately, I see athletes who, after reading one article or hearing an anecdotal report from a training partner or coach, mistakenly believe they should complete all training sessions in this low-carbohydrate state. These athletes are undoubtedly doing their bodies and performance a disservice, especially if these athletes are Masters athletes whose recovery nutrition is paramount to maintaining muscle mass and training load.

Athletes and coaches interested in experimenting with a higher-fat diet to fuel training should read all available research, consider each individual athlete's particular training and adaptation needs relative to training phase, nutrition and muscle mass goals, as well as duration of competition and availability of food or nutrition during competition. Adjustments should be made based on recovery and response to this strategy before proceeding to the potential detriment of the athlete's health and performance.

High-Fat and Ketogenic Diets for Masters Athletes: Fad or Functional?

As a registered dietitian, I first learned about and implemented ketogenic diets in the pediatric hospital in which I worked in New York City around 2000. We implemented them for children with severe seizure disorders, and for those whom the diets helped, the difficulty in maintaining such a strict regime was worth it. For those whom it did not help, the diet was abandoned due to both difficulty in implementing and risk of inadequacies in many key vitamins, minerals, and nutrients.

A few years later, when I started my private practice as a registered dietitian, I began seeing more people follow these high-fat diets for reasons including intended weight loss and a possible energy boost. Let's dig into the science of those trends now.

Traditional ketogenic diets involve careful planning and high dietary fat intake, generally with a four-to-one fat-to-protein or fat-to-carbohydrate ratio and a limit of 50 to 80 grams of total carbohydrate per day. (This is equal to that found in 1/2 cup nuts, 1 cup cooked broccoli, 1 cup cooked spinach, and 1 small piece of fruit.) There is an adaptation period during which fat oxidation increases; this phase can take weeks to months. Thereafter the results on athletic performance are unclear at best. The diet has been shown to cause athletes to become acutely catabolic, meaning their bodies are forced to break down muscle in order to supply adequate substrate to fuel their exercise demands. Negative symptoms widely reported include fatigue, headaches, poor concentration, gastrointestinal discomfort, lethargy, nausea, immunosuppression, and decreased lean body mass (Tiller et al. 2019), none of which sound advantageous to training or moving happily through our daily lives. Additionally, ketogenic diets are also low in fiber (thus the gastrointestinal distress), iron, magnesium, potassium, folate, and other important nutrients that are essential to athletes and for which athletes have higher needs than the general population. A ketogenic diet is particularly unhelpful for ultramarathon runners, who have previously been shown to have decreased intakes of important vitamins and minerals including magnesium and B-vitamins, and are recommended to follow a "mineral-rich approach involving plant-based foods and whole grains" in order to support overall training, energy, and health need (Tiller et al. 2019, page 17).

The bottom line here, after parsing through all available literature as of the writing of this book in 2020, is that while higher fat diets and training with higher fat (and thus lower carb) intake may lead to increased fat oxidation, it does not specifically lead to favorable changes in body composition and has been widely shown to decrease ability to perform at higher intensities (Tiller et al. 2019). To date, there has been no scientific evidence of any ergogenic effect of high-fat or ketogenic diets when compared to moderate- or high-carbohydrate diets in athletes.

Spotlight on Erica Agran

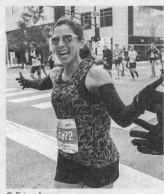

© Erica Agran

Erica Agran is a runner and fitness blogger who has run more than 400 races, 52 marathons, and over 150 half-marathons. She has run the New York City Marathon 20 times, thus earning herself guaranteed entry to the iconic race for life. She lives, trains, and connects people to other people and great things in Chicago, and she runs more miles each year than she drives. Erica's blog, www.EricaFinds.com, and social media sites (@EricaAgran) have more than 20,000 loyal followers who count on her for fitness ideas, products, and connections.

Erica and I met more than 20 years ago, not surprisingly, through running. We ran the New York City Marathon together in 2011, eight months after I gave birth to my third child and the year she survived a blood clot in her leg. We have traveled together to Zion National Park, the Grand Canyon, and Colorado to run, attend food shows and running retreats, and to explore, laugh, and taste healthy foods together.

How have you changed your nutritional intake as a Masters runner?

When I was younger, I really didn't pay attention to what I ate at all, but over time that has, of course, shifted. I have also found that we really need to listen to our changing bodies as we age. I had been training, racing, and traveling nonstop for years and feeling great. But we athletes often take on a lot—work, family obligations, training, travel—and it all leads to increased stress. Then, at 39, I had to take extended time off for a blood clot in my leg, and came back feeling better and running stronger. That forced time off taught me the true importance of rest and recovery, helped me to decrease my cortisol, and really recover my body from the prior years of training. I also take more vitamins and supplements on a daily basis now than I did when I was younger. At age 43 or 44 I was no longer feeling like my usual self. My energy plummeted, my performance was suffering, and my weight was creeping up. I never really felt rested and was dealing with what felt like a lot of inflammation. A lot of people said, "You are just getting older," and of course we are all getting older, but I felt that wasn't really the whole problem.

I started seeing a naturopathic doctor and taking adaptogens and other vitamins. Pretty shortly thereafter I started feeling better, and my performance improved again. Finally, when I was younger I used to think I had to give up alcohol and caffeine for a month before each marathon, but as I have gotten older, I realize that a glass of wine or cup of coffee is not going to hurt me or adversely affect anything. I enjoy my coffee, and now I find that enjoying a glass of wine can be a nice way to relax the night before a marathon. So that is a big change for me.

Have you changed your intake of any macronutrient as a Masters athlete?

Yes! In my early 40s I started experimenting with eating more nuts and nut butters, which I had previously not eaten much of due to growing up at a time when fat-free foods were the craze. As I added the higher fat foods, I started to notice that my energy was better, my weight was stable, and I felt better overall. I have the amazing opportunity to meet (and run with) so many athletes, and specifically female runners, because I travel for my blog, speak to groups, and serve as an ambassador for many products and races. One of the problems as I see it is that so many female athletes are scared of food. After years of hearing conflicting information on which foods are "bad" for them, they are severely limiting their variety of food. This is really sad because it should be all about balance. If you want to give me a bar of dark chocolate and container of cashew nuts any day, I say, "Bring it on." And because I eat these real and filling foods, including higher fat foods, I feel full and satisfied. I always had a sweet tooth, and now that I eat more foods that are naturally high in fat, I really don't crave sweets the way I used to.

What is your inside perspective on the changing world of nutrition products?

I go to all the healthy food and fitness expos across the country each year and have seen a huge increase in the number of functional food products, which makes it more confusing for people to figure out what they should really be putting into their bodies. It is really interesting how food trends shift drastically. When I was in college we thought low-fat was the way to go. We were kids of the low-fat craze. Back then, no one seemed to care about whether they were eating wholesome, real food; they only cared whether it was low fat. I would never have eaten real salad dressing or nut butters back then. Now I make real salad dressing with different oils; use nuts, seeds, and avocado in salads; and put nut butters in oatmeal, on apples, or eat them straight from the jar. I also used to use skim milk and dairy and now would never tell anyone to do that. One big promising nutrition and health trend is that a large percentage of people are looking for real food, and because of that there are more real food bars, snacks, and truly healthy foods at each food show I attend and on the shelves. But at the same time, we have to be aware. There are many "natural" food companies that write to me, asking me to review or promote their "healthy" products and touting that they have zero carbs and zero sugar. But what is in them? Many of them are not real food, and that is not healthy. That is not what I, or any of us, should be interested in.

Do you have any nutritional words of wisdom to share with us?

First, make the switch to real foods. Try cutting out some or all of the fake, low-fat products for one or two weeks and see if you feel less hungry and if your running feels easier. Whatever it is you are looking to change, does it improve when eating more real, full-fat foods? Second, know what your goals are. Right now, my athletic goals are to continue running and traveling as long as it is fun and feels good. I have made hundreds of friends across the country through running and have people I love to run with anywhere I could possibly want to go.

Erica's Favorite Postrace Meal

Fried chicken or a big burger followed by a black and white cookie (especially if I am in New York City). These are three foods I normally eat only after running long distances.

If you do want to try some higher fat intake fueling during training, keep it to workouts where you are working at less than 70 percent of your $\dot{V}O_2$max, when gastric emptying rates are less impeded; you should still be able to digest these traditionally slower-digesting foods. Many ultramarathon runners are likely thinking, "I do that already!" And yes, since running ultras are performed at less than 70 percent $\dot{V}O_2$max in order to continue moving forward for that prolonged duration of time, these athletes tend to do best with higher calorie and higher overall fat intakes during these grueling events.

Supporting what our best ultraendurance athletes have already come to know, the International Society of Sports Nutrition (ISSN) recommends 150 to 300 calories per hour for races up to 50 miles, and 200 to 400 calories per hour for longer races (Kerksick et al. 2018). Studies specifically show that endurance athletes who take in less than 200 calories per hour have a higher rate of noncompletion and that finishers of 100-mile races consume an average of five times more total fat during the race or run than nonfinishers, suggesting a need for higher total calories and total fat. They have also shown two times the total carbohydrate intake of non-finishers and an average of 333 calories per hour (Tiller et al. 2019). A higher fat intake may be warranted and critical to the success of ultraendurance athletes, especially because fat provides more energy (calories) per gram, which helps athletes maintain that critical high-calorie, high-energy intake during these endurance events that can take at least 10 to 13 hours. That said, carbohydrate is clearly not to be overlooked, because it continues to provide an integral fuel source necessary for both race completion as well as maintaining cognitive function and endurance performance (Tiller et al. 2019).

One important final note is that there seems to be a high degree of individual variability in capacity to switch between carbohydrate oxidation and fat oxidation at absolute workloads. This means that each of us is an experiment of one, and we need to note what feels and works best to us, not blindly follow what other athletes, coaches, or studies say worked for them.

In chapter 8, we discuss many of the popular supplements athletes want to know about and get to the bottom of which ones might be worth trying and for whom.

8 | Supplements

Supplements are a huge business among athletes and nonathletes alike. People want to look, feel, and perform their best, and often seek out quick fixes or additional ways to get ahead in addition to, or sometimes instead of, a healthy diet and regular exercise. In fact, according to the 2018 Council for Responsible Nutrition (CRN) consumer survey on dietary supplements, 75 percent of U.S. adults report taking a supplement on a regular basis, and of those, 70 percent report exercising regularly. The survey also reports that the number of U.S. adults using supplements has increased by 10 percent since 2009 and now includes 78 percent of U.S. adults over age 55 and 77 percent of U.S. adults ages 35 to 54. To be clear, supplements can include not only vitamins or minerals, but also functional foods (foods that have vitamins or minerals added directly into them); sports foods; and a wide assortment of pills, capsules, and powders. Neither annual income nor education level influences a person's likelihood of using dietary supplements, but age certainly does. At least three out of four of you reading this book are likely taking supplements as part of your regular routine.

The number-one reported reason for adults over the age of 35 to be taking a supplement is overall health and wellness. Energy, bone health, and nutrient gaps also ranked high as reasons for taking supplements. Multivitamin use was reported by 83 percent of those ages 18 to 34, 75 percent among 35- to 54-year-olds, and 70 percent among adults 55 years and older (CRN 2018). As we get older, we tend to choose specific supplements rather than a good old-fashioned multivitamin. A multivitamin is still the most popular choice, followed by vitamin D, then protein, calcium, vitamin C, and B vitamins. The report also found that in general, 87 percent of U.S. adults say they have confidence in the safety, quality, and effectiveness of supplements they are buying. This statistic is quite interesting, considering that supplement sales in the U.S. often precede adequate scientific research of the claims made by companies trying to sell you their product.

In this chapter I will present you with the latest scientific research on many of the most popular and noteworthy supplements taken by athletes. We will focus mostly on the ones that have been shown to work, and I will delineate which athletes might benefit from each, and how. Included in this supplement review are caffeine, creatine, nitrate or beetroot, sodium bicarbonate, and beta-alanine, which currently show the most promise in terms of enhancing athletic performance. I will also present information to help you decide if you should take a multivitamin, iron, calcium, vitamin D, curcumin and turmeric, collagen, melatonin, and others.

It may be helpful to understand the research process. The gold standard for research studies, including those investigating the effects of supplements, are double blind, randomized, controlled scientific trials, which are then reported in peer-reviewed scientific journals. These studies are most reliable because they test individuals receiving a supplement against individuals receiving a placebo (a known substance that has no therapeutic effect), which is used as a control by which to test the difference. Using a placebo helps keep both the scientists and participants blind to which participants are receiving the supplements. Good studies also use a large enough sample size to be considered reliable; use a crossover design (i.e., all participants will be tested after receiving the supplement and after receiving only the placebo); are repeatable by other scientists; and have real-life benefit. Important things to consider when evaluating the validity of a study include whether the researchers controlled for dietary intake; whether total calories, protein, or other macronutrient intake changed under the experimental conditions; and whether the testing conditions are typical for an athlete. For example, did participants eat their usual breakfast with the prerace supplement?

It is important to keep in mind that blog posts, advertisements, and social media posts are not substitutes for true scientific research data and are not monitored for accuracy in content. Therefore, beware—only you are responsible for what you decide to buy and put into your body. Supplements sold in the United States are not regulated by the government (in the United States, by the Food and Drug Administration [FDA]) as they are in some other countries. Once they are already on the market for the public to buy and ingest, the FDA can recall any product that contains more of an ingredient than is listed, is likely to have a toxicity risk, or is contaminated with ingredients not intended to be in the product that may be harmful to an individual, including lead and glass (Maughan et al. 2018). However, someone has to bring it to the FDA's attention in order for a recall to occur. In 2015 it was estimated that 23,000 trips to the emergency room resulted from use of supplements that were either taken in excess or in combination with other supplements, thus leading to adverse effects.

Athletes' responsibility for what they ingest includes medications given to or prescribed by a doctor as well as any over-the-counter medications, supplements, or creams. Athletes who compete at a national or international level are responsible for knowing the list of prohibited substances and methods and for cooperating with sample collection as requested. The World Anti-Doping Agency (WADA) states that their mission is to lead a collaborative worldwide movement for doping-free sport. They have a core document that athletes and coaches should review to ensure familiarity with their policies and responsibilities. For the rest of us nonelite athletes, we too should want to know what we are putting into our bodies.

While it might be important to correct a vitamin or nutrient deficiency, taking certain supplements without first having your lab values checked and knowing your numbers can lead to overdose. This is especially true for iron and fat-soluble vitamins that are not excreted through urine and thus build up in your body when taken in excess. I caution you to supplement only if and when you are certain you have deficiencies, to follow recommended doses and duration of supplementation, and to ensure you have done your research into any product's efficacy and ingredients before you begin taking anything. While it is sometimes true that even a small performance improvement can make a big difference in the outcome of your game, race, or season, check for third-party certification. NSF International conducts third-party testing and provides certification for products and supplements. The NSF Certified Sport mark means that NSF International has tested the product and verified that it is free from contaminants, does not contain any hidden ingredients, contains what it states it contains, and does not contain any athletic-banned substances in the product or its ingredients. This certification is recognized by the NFL, MLB, PGA, and other major sports organizations. However, NSF does not certify efficacy (i.e., it does not test whether the product actually does what is claims it will do). In this chapter we will discuss how to do this research. But first, we now turn to an NFL linebacker who had an impressive 10-year professional American football career and who attributes his longevity in this strenuous sport to good nutrition and smart (but not excessive) supplementation.

Prevalence of Nutritional Supplementation

According to the International Olympic Committee (IOC) consensus statement on dietary supplements and the high-performance athlete (Maughan et al. 2018), adult athletes are likely to report taking supplements in an attempt to increase lean body mass (LMB), decrease fat mass, or increase their performance. (As discussed in chapter 6, adequate protein intake is one of the best ways to preserve LMB and decrease fat mass [Maughan et al. 2018], especially as we age.) At the highest level of athletic competition, a 1 percent increase in performance, ranging from 45 seconds to 8 minutes, can affect the medal rankings (Christensen et al. 2017), so athletes might

Spotlight on Connor Barwin

Connor Barwin was an outside linebacker in the NFL for 10 years. He attended and played football at the University of Cincinnati, was drafted by the Houston Texans in the second round in 2009, played four years in Houston, four years for the Philadelphia Eagles, one year for the Los Angeles Rams, and, finally, a year for the New York Giants. Connor also started the Make the World Better Foundation (MTWB.org), which "connects people and inspires stewardship through public space revitalization projects." He credits changing his nutrition to his ability to recover well and to his longevity in his high-impact sport.

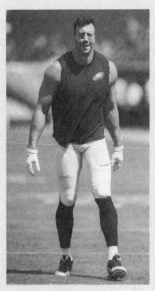

Mitchell Leff/Getty Images

What are you most proud of in terms of your athletic career?

I am most proud of my ability to stay healthy. After I broke my ankle during the first game of my second year in Houston and missed the whole season, I came back the next year and went on to start about 120 games in six straight seasons. I never missed a game or a snap. In the NFL, they say availability is stability. I was really proud that I was consistently available for my team, and I strongly believe that my nutrition played a large role in that.

How has your nutritional intake shifted throughout your career?

For me specifically, as a linebacker graduating college and entering the NFL, I initially had to gain weight. I was drinking a ton of milk, eating lots of peanut butter and jelly sandwiches, and consuming as much protein and protein supplements with a ton of added sugar as I could. We ate anything and everything; mainly a lot of processed food and sugar. I think this is a consistent problem for athletes expending a lot of calories. How can I get in the food and calories I need in a quality way? Those foods definitely helped us put on weight, but most of those foods are things that I would not eat now. As I got a little older, I still needed to take in enough calories, but I started choosing more good calories—more fish, different types of pasta plus beans. I also shifted to real, homemade smoothies two or three times a day. I still got enough sugar (carbs) from the fruits in there, and I was able to include tons of veggies plus chia seeds or oats or anything I could find that I was being told was good for me. It all went into the smoothies.

During the second half of my career playing in the NFL, I reduced the amount of sugar in my diet and focused on reducing inflammation. In football, as you well know, we were always sore, and anything we could do to recover faster and decrease the inflammation made a big difference. Changing my nutrition for the better while still playing in the NFL definitely had a positive impact on my career. I have no doubt about that. But those shifts have made an even bigger difference in terms of how I feel now postcareer, because I still feel pretty good. And those choices will continue to pay off for the rest of my life.

What types of supplements have you taken throughout your career?

There's a range of supplements the players in the NFL take, and for the first five or six years of my career, I took a lot: one before my workout, a protein powder, one after my workout, one before sleep—five or six bottles of "stuff" each day. Then, when I got to Philly, I started asking myself what I should be eating in the morning to fuel me before practice. What was the best thing to eat after practice? I also realized I was probably eating too much protein. I would drink several different protein shakes throughout the day, and I would also have to run to the bathroom all day. Looking back, let's say that when your intestines aren't operating normally, that is a sign that you're probably eating too much of something. Another major shift I made was that during the last three to four years of my professional career, I started taking a product called MEND Orthopedic for recovery. It has whey protein—specifically, leucine and glutamine—and also turmeric, iron, and vitamin C. My strength coach initially told me to try it, and I loved it immediately. I started taking MEND first thing when I woke up in the morning and last thing at night. I loved how it made me feel, and I know that it really helped me survive the wear and tear my body had to absorb through each season. Since then, I take only this one supplement, and I definitely feel better. MEND plus some coffee or caffeine are all I have taken from then on, and I still use it today.

How have you seen the conversation regarding nutrition shift within the NFL?

Thankfully, there's been a major shift in the NFL in terms of thinking about nutrition over the last 12 to 15 years. When I started to play for the Eagles, the coach brought in a whole big sports science team, which was really a cultural shift in the NFL. From then on, there was a lot more focus on nutrition and diet as well as sleep and hydration, things we all knew were important but had not always prioritized. He put processes in place within the team that made it easier for us to get the foods we needed and to get the right supplements. We started working with nutritionists, and they started making us each a custom smoothie that contained different amounts of protein, carbs, and sugars relative to what each of our goals were.

Many athletes, especially in football since it's such a physically demanding sport, after a few years of playing at the highest level have to start eating better to feel better. You start to realize that the foods you eat make a big difference, especially in your recovery. Now I believe every team has at least one sport nutritionist, and they don't give out anti-inflammatory medications or painkillers like they did 15 to 20 years ago. Now the first intervention is nutrition. And, you and I both know that nutrition makes a huge difference.

Connor's Favorite Postgame Meal

You are not going to like this, but I would usually order pizza after every game.*

* I am not sure why so many athletes feel the need to preface this answer with "you are not going to like this," but by now you should realize that I am a huge believer in all foods fitting into our lives, as well as the importance of enjoying our foods while we fuel our performance, recovery, and health. Three cheers for postgame pizza.

look for any small improvements through legal and ethical supplementation. We will now focus on supplements that might serve to improve an athlete's performance directly or may facilitate recovery after exercise.

The Australian Institute of Sport (AIS) has classified sport supplements into categories by scientific, evidence-based, and performance effects. Class A supplements are those considered to have a high level of evidence to support their use in improving athletic performance. We will start by reviewing those five supplements, which include caffeine, creatine, nitrate or beetroot juice, beta-alanine, and sodium bicarbonate.

Caffeine

Caffeine is a substance with which most of us are very familiar; 90 percent of us consume it regularly (Nehlig 2018) and can attest to its benefits. Caffeine is derived from cocoa beans, tea leaves, and some nuts, and is widely accepted and consumed around the globe by billions of people daily, mainly in the form of coffee (71%) and tea (12%), as well as sport drinks and other sport products. The average intake of caffeine is just over 200 milligrams per day, which can be found in about 16 ounces of coffee (Nehlig 2018).

Do you really know why you like your daily caffeine fix or why many of us take it before or during exercise? Caffeine works in the brain to increase arousal, decrease rate of perceived exertion (RPE), and decrease muscle pain, all of which help inspire us to get or keep moving. Even small doses can lead to an increased feeling of alertness and a boost to your motivation to work out and to overall performance.

It has been well established that caffeine use by athletes improves exercise performance across a broad range of activities, including aerobic endurance, muscle strength, muscular endurance power, jumping performance, and speed or sprinting (Anderson et al. 2000). The 2018 IOC published a consensus statement regarding caffeine use in athletes (Maughan et al. 2018), in which they stated that 74 percent of urine samples they collected for doping control from 2004 to 2008 contained caffeine. Although caffeine was once banned by the IOC and WADA, it no longer is.

The good news for Masters athletes is that it works for athletes of all ages. Studies have demonstrated a 25 percent increase in cycling performance, 54 percent increase in arm flexion endurance, and decreased RPE in adults older than 70 years after ingestion of 6 milligrams per kilogram of body weight of caffeine (about 12 to 16 oz of regular coffee) prior to exercise (Tallis et al. 2013). Additionally, caffeine intake has been shown to improve mood as well as psychological and cognitive performance in older adults (Tallis et al. 2013), which may be due to its ability to increase activation in the central nervous system. When given 3 milligrams per kilogram of body weight versus a placebo 60 minutes prior to exercise, caffeine supplementation was shown to significantly improve mood state by 17 percent, decrease error rate in timing tasks by 35 percent, and increase muscular strength in older adults.

The typical tested dose ranges from 3 to 6 milligrams per kilogram of body weight and is generally taken about 60 minutes prior to the start of the activity. Caffeine is known to be rapidly absorbed in the gastrointestinal tract with peak concentration after about 30 minutes and full absorption within 45 minutes of ingestion. Its effects are not dependent on age or sex (Nehlig 2018). Studies have shown additional benefit and improved performance when both caffeine and carbohydrate are consumed before and during exercise (Maughan et al. 2018). Studies also have consistently shown that caffeine increases endurance performance for exercise lasting 20 to 250 minutes by increasing exercise time to fatigue, and caffeine improved time trial performance by 3 to 7 percent in activities including cycling, running, and rowing (Maughan et al. 2018). Furthermore, taking 100 to 300 milligrams of caffeine 15 to 80 minutes into endurance exercise further improves cycling performance by 3 to 7 percent (Maughan et al. 2018).

For sprinters, some studies have shown that taking 3 to 6 milligrams per kilogram of body weight of caffeine 50 to 60 minutes prior to short-sprint activities can increase power output, task completion time, and repeat sprint performance lasting one to two minutes by 3 percent. However, study results are mixed on caffeine's effects for short-duration exercise (i.e., activities lasting 45 seconds to 20 minutes) (Christensen et al. 2017). As such, more studies are needed. See table 8.1 for your optimal exercise caffeine dose by body weight.

As with physical training, more is not always better. Doses higher than 9 milligrams per kilogram of body weight do not show increased performance benefit, but rather serve only to increase the risk of side effects including nausea, anxiety, insomnia, and restlessness.

Athletes who consume caffeine daily may be wondering how habituation affects caffeine's performance-enhancing effects. Conventional wisdom is that low-habitual caffeine users will experience a larger ergogenic effect versus high-habitual caffeine users. However, studies have not found this to be the case (Grgic et al. 2019). Many factors may be at play here, including method of caffeine delivery (caffeine pills, coffee or tea, energy gels or chews), as well as duration of time between caffeine consumption and start of exercise bout. More studies are needed to further our knowledge in this area.

TABLE 8.1   Caffeine Dose by Athlete Weight

Caffeine dose	120 lb (54 kg) athlete	160 lb (73 kg) athlete	200 lb (91 kg) athlete
3 mg/kg (1 mg/lb) body weight	163 mg	218 mg	272 mg
6 mg/kg (3 mg/lb) body weight	327 mg	436 mg	545 mg

Note that a typical 8-ounce cup of coffee contains about 100 milligrams of caffeine, so 16 ounces of coffee taken one hour prior to exercise would provide about 200 milligrams. A cup of white or green tea generally contains 25 to 40 milligrams of caffeine, and black and oolong tea can contain 50 to 75 milligrams of caffeine per cup.

Spotlight on Jackie Edwards-Flowers

Jackie Edwards-Flowers is a five-time Olympic long jumper. She competed for Stanford University, then had an impressive Olympic career spanning from age 21 (Barcelona in 1992) to age 37 (Beijing in 2008). Jackie attributes her longevity in sport to good genetics that allowed her to train continually and her intrinsic motivation to be the best she can at whatever she does. She is a testament to what you can achieve when you put your mind to it.

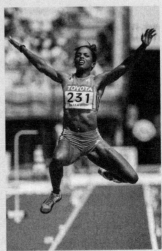

Mitchell Leff/Getty Images

How would you describe your overall nutrition philosophy?

I was always mindful about what I ate and tried to cut down on sugar over the years, but everything else was fair game. I always wanted to be fueled, and I also have low blood sugar at times, so I never skipped breakfast. I ate a bowl of cereal or a bagel every single day. I definitely ate carbs, not because someone told me to, but because I felt good eating them and after eating them. Now that I'm a "civilian" who exercises two or three times a week, I have certainly changed how much I eat and have decreased my refined carb intake. When I am coaching an athlete or a team, or when a friend introduces me as "My friend who competed in the Olympics five times," I never want anyone to look at me incredulously. It is my way of motivating myself to stay healthy and reasonably fit.

What was your nutritional transition like in college and beyond?

In college I was left on my own for nutrition, which as it turned out, was not a good thing. Having been born in Jamaica and growing up in the Bahamas, I ate Jamaican food, all the while not having any idea or appreciation that Jamaican food is generally healthy. It is all from the ground or from an animal. Everything was homemade, broiled, baked, stewed, or grilled. I got to college with no understanding of what I should be eating, and within three months I gained 25 pounds. Sure, I was lifting weights and I put on muscle quickly, but I was also not eating well. Combine those two factors, and the physics of that did not work out; as a long jumper I needed to fly through the air. I was yelled and screamed at about my weight every day for two years, and I cried every other day. It was not good, but I also knew I had to figure it out, because I could not call my parents and tell them that I could not keep my scholarship at Stanford because I could not figure out my nutrition. I first went to a dietitian freshman year. I was skipping meals, and she told me to eat more. I remember thinking, "This woman is not listening to me. I am trying to lose weight, and she keeps telling me to eat more." I didn't understand that she meant I needed to eat more regular meals and more times during the day, so I ignored everything she said. But skipping meals obviously didn't work, so I kept putting on weight. After my sophomore year, my coach told me that if I didn't lose weight over the summer I could come back to class junior year but not to track practice—and he was serious. I went to the dietitian again, and again she told me to eat more. This time I thought, "Well, I have tried everything else, so maybe she is correct." I did everything she said, and—surprise—it worked! I lost the weight by eating more good food and doing regular exercise, nothing crazy. I finally understood how it all worked and what my body needed.

How did you deal psychologically with your coach's weight ultimatum?

It was not good for a while, and many of the girls quit because there was a lot of language that you just had to figure out how to handle.

Making five Olympic teams is no easy feat. What were the keys to your continued success?

If you can stay healthy, you can maintain your level of fitness and improve from there. I went from not qualifying for NCAA championships my first two years of college to being second in my junior year, and then NCAA champion by my senior year. Throughout my career I saw athletes take steroids and then become better than me, and others quit not believing they could compete without taking what the others were taking. But I never gave up or gave in. I knew I couldn't change what anyone else was doing, so I stayed in it for myself and found great satisfaction in improving myself. For me, taking performance-enhancing drugs was never an option. Achieving something knowing I didn't achieve it all by myself—where is the joy in that?

Did you ever take any nutritional supplements?

Most definitely. I worked with world renowned coach Dan Pfaff for five years. His knowledge in everything from coaching to biomechanics to nutrition to injury to supplementation is second to none. Under his coaching, I took L-glutamine, glucosamine and chondroitin, L-arginine, L-ornithine, L-carnitine, a multivitamin, and vitamin C. Many of the athletes also took creatine, but I skipped that one because I was always very muscular and didn't need to gain muscle or deal with the side effects of water retention or cramping. I also typically consumed a caffeinated drink before intense jumping workouts and competitions.

How have your nutrition and recovery shifted as a Masters athlete?

Relative to when I competed, people may think I look the same, but I am probably 12 to 15 pounds heavier now. I am mindful but also realistic about what I eat. I don't avoid anything. I always bring a snack bag with me, which contains cheese, carrots, nuts, fruits, salami, yogurts, and granola bars, and I generally eat four or five of those while we are out. Everyone laughs at me—until they ask me for one of my snacks! I am a mom to three boys, and we have a lot of kid food in our house. I am mindful not to eat their food. Later in my career I also started taking an extra day off during the week, which really helped with recovery. I realized that it is 10 times more important to be healthy than worry about not training one day. You have to be diligent and committed and consistent, but when your body tells you it is tired, you need to listen.

Jackie's Favorite Postcompetition Meal

My postcompetition meal varied depending on the country I was in, and more important than what I would eat, was the relaxation and enjoyment I felt after a competition. Therefore, I would usually eat multiple courses: appetizer, meal, and dessert.

Another area of research on caffeine intake and metabolism is the effect of the menstrual cycle phase and hormonal shifts on the metabolism and elimination of caffeine. Lane et al. (1992) found evidence to suggest that caffeine elimination may be slower during the late luteal phase, just prior to the onset of menstruation. More recent investigations (Nehlig 2018) explained how estrogen competes for inhibitors of caffeine metabolism, which may explain the effect of slower caffeine elimination during the late luteal phase, but the significance of this effect is not yet known.

Creatine

Creatine is a nitrogenous organic compound that is found in muscle tissue and stored in fast-twitch type II muscle in humans and other animals and can be found (and ingested) mainly in milk, red meat, and fish. Typical carnivores get about 1 to 2 grams of creatine per day in their diets.

This popular sport nutrition supplement is often used in an effort to increase LBM, muscle mass, and muscle strength, and has most recently seen $400 million in annual supplement sales (Butts, Jacobs, and Silvis 2017). Creatine loading has been shown to acutely enhance performance in high-intensity exercise involving repeated movements such as in team sports, as well as resistance and interval training regimes (Maughan et al. 2018). Studies have also shown that creatine supplementation, beginning with a loading phase of about 20 grams per day (divided equally into four doses spread throughout the day) for five to seven days leads to increased lean muscle mass, strength, and power. After the loading phase, one goes into a maintenance phase and takes 3 to 5 grams per day in a single dose for the duration of the supplementation cycle. As with caffeine, further gains were noted when creatine was taken along with substrate (i.e., food), which helps increase creatine uptake via increased insulin secretion. In this case, creatine was taken with a source containing about 50 grams of protein and carbohydrate together. It is worth noting that the most pronounced effects were seen in exercises lasting less than 30 seconds and next in those lasting less than 150 seconds (2.5 minutes). A limited number of studies have also found improved endurance performance as a result of increased protein synthesis, glycogen storage, and thermoregulation (Maughan et al. 2018), but it seems most effective for short-duration, maximum-intensity sports.

Determining the adequate but not excessive amount you should take it is not straightforward. Studies have demonstrated results with varying doses and when taken for varied durations of time. Some have used 0.7 grams per kilogram of body weight for five days, while others, including the International Society of Sports Nutrition, recommend a more gradual 0.3 grams per kilogram of body weight (Butts, Jacobs, and Silvis 2017). In terms of duration of supplementation, studies have looked at supplementation effects after as short as three days of loading and up to four to six weeks (Butts,

Jacobs, and Silvis 2017). Additionally, wide variation in responses has been noted among athletes even within the same protocol and sport, which are likely due to differences in starting levels of creatine in athlete's bodies due to previous dietary intake. Overall, 64 percent of creatine studies examined showed an increase in LBM as well as water retention and decreased urine production due to fluid shifts when creatine is ingested and stored (Butts, Jacobs, and Silvis 2017). Bigger effects were seen in terms of increased strength, muscular power, and one-rep maximum in previously untrained individuals, so those of us who have been training for years might not reap as many benefits from this popular supplement.

Two creatine dosing options exist. The first dosing option is based on body weight: you would ingest 0.3 grams of creatine per kilogram of body weight for three days for four to six weeks. That would be 16 grams per day for a 120-pound (54 kg) athlete, 22 grams per day for a 160-pound (73 kg) athlete, and 27 grams per day for a 200-pound (91 kg) athlete. The second dosing option is ingestion of 20 grams per day, regardless of body weight, during a week-long loading phase, then 3 to 5 grams per day for maintenance.

Some studies have found improved recovery as well as increased LBM and strength following a disuse injury when creatine is taken (Maughan et al. 2018). Athletes might benefit from creatine supplementation when recovering from injury or surgery, but additional studies are needed.

To date, when loading and maintenance protocols have been followed, no negative health consequences have been noted with long-term use (up to four years), though more long-term studies are needed to continue to test for any longer-term effects. Many athletes will note a 1- to 2-kilogram increase in total body weight as a result of water retention associated with creatine supplementation. This would be disadvantageous for many athletes, including jumpers and pole vaulters who need to fly up in the sky, athletes in weight classification sports, or those who are trying to achieve specific power-to-weight ratios for performance purposes.

As with most supplements, products containing creatine are not screened for banned substances by WADA, IOC, or NCAA, and are not regulated by the USDA; therefore, the athlete assumes all risk of taking any supplement and knowing what is inside any product, whether it is written on the label or might be contaminated with something that is not listed on the label (Butts, Jacobs, and Silvis 2017).

Nitrate and Beetroot

Nitrate is another popular supplement that has been shown to improve performance by enhancing type II muscle fiber function and improving blood flow to muscles in some athletes. One study showed improved performance when a single dose of 5 to 9 millimoles (310-560 mg) of nitrate was given two to three hours prior to exercise (Maughan et al. 2018), while other three-day protocols have also shown promise. Study protocols and results vary widely in the performance effects found. Some have shown improved exercise time to exhaustion by 4 to 25 percent and improved sport-specific time trial performance lasting less than 40 minutes by 1 to 3 percent (Maughan et al. 2018). Others demonstrate an improvement in high-intensity, intermittent team-sport performance lasting 12 to 40 minutes in duration (Maughan et al. 2018). Initial studies have shown little benefit for exercise lasting less than 12 minutes or for prolonged endurance performance (Maughan et al. 2018).

Beetroot contains dietary nitrate (NO_3-) and has been proven to increase blood concentrations of nitric oxide (NO), leading to increased blood flow to muscles and increased vasodilation (Domínguez et al. 2018). Beetroot supplementation has shown promise for explosive efforts lasting less than six seconds, high-intensity efforts lasting between six seconds and one minute, and also for intense exercise lasting greater than 60 minutes (Domínguez et al. 2018).

Overall, results of supplementation are often not straightforward, as is exemplified by the fact that in one recent review of beetroot, four studies showed performance improvement while four others showed no effect (Domínguez et al. 2018). The positive studies have shown the potential for beetroot supplementation to increase cycling ergometer performance in tests to exhaustion at 60 to 90 percent maximum intensity ($\dot{V}O_2$max) by 12 to 17 percent, improve performance at 70 percent $\dot{V}O_2$max by 22 percent, and increase performance in trained cyclists over distances ranging from 4 kilometers (2 mi, 2.8% improvement), 10 kilometers (6 mi, 1.2%), 16 kilometers (10 mi, 2.7%), and 50 miles (80 km, 0.8%) when beetroot was taken 120 minutes before exercise for 5 to 7 days (Dominguez et al. 2018). As you will find when you scientifically review most supplements, more research is needed to help delineate which duration of exercise can be most affected by nitrate and beetroot supplementation. Also, as with many supplements studied, it is difficult to control for all variables in order to get clear-cut and universally consistent results.

Beetroot does not seem to help endurance performance in highly trained individuals (defined as $\dot{V}O_2$max higher than 70 mL/kg), because they generally already have a high endogenous capacity for NO production (Christensen et al. 2017). But once again, there seem to be responders and nonresponders, noted by wide individual variation in performance improvement following supplementation even among trained individuals. As with other supplements, studies show a smaller effect in highly trained athletes, reinforcing the plethora of beneficial effects our bodies are capable of just by training consistently. As always, there is an upper limit to what nitrate supplementation can do; no greater benefit has been seen when taking 16.8 millimoles (104 mg) versus 8.4 millimoles (521 mg) (Maughan et al. 2018).

If you feel that your exercise duration and type falls into a range that might make it worth experimenting with beetroot, first try boosting your blood flow and performance by adding food sources high in nitrates into your usual dietary intake. These include leafy greens, citrus, garlic, root vegetables (e.g., spinach, celery, and beets), and dark chocolate. For athletes engaging in intermittent, maximum-intensity, short-duration explosive efforts lasting 6 to 10 seconds, with brief bouts of recovery (less than 30 seconds), beetroot juice supplementation might be worth a try, because it could help your body more rapidly replace phosphocreatine reserves to avoid depletion and thus allow better results on later sets. It might also help to decrease muscular fatigue associated with high-intensity efforts and associated muscle damage (Domínguez et al. 2018). However, if either your work time or recovery time is longer, you might want to look elsewhere or simply train harder and smarter to get the results you desire. Evidence shows a small potential for gastrointestinal upset in some athletes taking nitrate, so as always, this and any supplementation should be tested many times in training before use on competition or race day.

Sodium Bicarbonate

Bicarbonate acts as a buffering agent in the bloodstream, and its supplementation has been shown to increase the pH of the blood by about 0.1, which may help to postpone fatigue during intense exercise, specifically in sustained high-intensity exercise lasting about 6 minutes, or possibly up to 10 minutes (Christensen et al. 2017). This effect is presumably attributable to decreasing acidosis experiences during intense exercise. A review article (Hadzic, Eckstein, and Schugardt 2019) analyzed the results of 35 studies. Among those 35 studies, they showed that 11 of the 20 studies looking at exercise lasting < 4 minutes in duration found a net positive effect of bicarbonate supplementation, and that 6 of the 15 studies looking at exercise lasting > 4 minutes (running, tennis, or taekwondo) demonstrated improvements in performances. Furthermore, 17 of the 35 studies showed enhancement in performance (up to 3%) for swimmers, boxers, runners, and cyclists for events lasting < 4 minutes .

A single dose of sodium bicarbonate ($NaHCO_3$) taken as 0.2 to 0.4 grams per kilogram of body weight 60 to 150 minutes prior to commencing exercise has been shown to be effective at enhancing short-term (about 60 seconds), high-intensity exercise performance by about 2 percent (Maughan et al. 2018). Other studies that used split doses adding up to the same supplementation range 30 to 180 minutes before exercise showed similar results (Maughan et al. 2018). A several-day protocol testing $NaHCO_3$ supplementation given as several smaller doses per day over the two to four days prior to performance testing show diverse results (Hadzic, Eckstein, and Schugardt 2019). Despite much promising research, the evidence is far from conclusive.

- Supplementing with bicarbonate and caffeine yields added performance benefits (Hadzic, Eckstein, and Schugardt 2019).

- Studies have failed to show similar effects for exercise longer than 10 minutes.
- Overall, less promising results have been demonstrated in better trained athletes, whose bodies seem to have already trained themselves to have a higher buffering capacity.
- There appear to be responders and nonresponders.
- Most studies have been done in men. Effects in women in general or during different phases of their menstrual cycle are unknown.

It's important to know that a high rate of gastrointestinal distress has consistently been reported among athletes taking $NaHCO_3$. If that does not deter you and you do short- to middle-distance, high-intensity competition (200 m swim, 4K bike, 1,500 m run), it is recommended that you experiment in training long before trying it before a competition. Consume the supplement with a carbohydrate-rich meal of about 1.5 grams per kilogram of body weight of carbohydrate (Maughan et al. 2018). Other strategies include using the small, split-dose method or supplementing with sodium citrate to help lessen the chances or severity of gastrointestinal distress.

Beta-Alanine

Beta-alanine is another intracellular buffering agent with the potential to help improve sustained high-intensity exercise performance (Maughan et al. 2018). Chronic daily supplementation with beta-alanine has been shown to increase skeletal muscle carnosine content, which is the rate-limiting precursor to this important buffering process (Maughan et al. 2018). Carnosine has been shown to play an integral role in exercise performance and can be obtained both by dietary sources (proteins including meat, fish, and turkey) and supplementation. Dosage recommendation is about 65 milligrams per kilogram of body weight, taken at 0.8 to 1.6 grams every three to four hours over a period of 10 to 12 weeks. At this dosage, studies show small increases (0.2-3%) in performance for both continuous and intermittent tasks lasting 30 seconds and possibly up to 10 minutes, with a maximum effect seen in exercise lasting one to four minutes. No effect has been seen in exercise lasting less than one minute or greater than 10 minutes (Saunders et al. 2017).

It should not come as a surprise that a large variation is seen in terms of performance improvement following beta-alanine supplementation and that more studies are needed, especially in well-trained athletes and across more sports. This was very clearly demonstrated in a 2017 review article (Saunders et al. 2017) that examined 40 studies on beta-alanine supplementation, in which over 65 exercise protocols were used and 70 exercises were studied. The researchers found a significant overall effect in terms of increased exercise capacity and possibly in improved exercise performance when supplementation of 3.2 to 6.4 grams per day were used for two to four weeks and exercise duration was 30 seconds to 10 minutes. They again pointed to a smaller effect in highly trained individuals, although as mentioned earlier, even seemingly very small performance enhancements can make a big difference in overall outcome at the highest level of competition. Of course, more studies are warranted on this, as in other supplements, to help athletes make informed decisions.

Now that we have reviewed the five supplements that have strong enough evidence to be considered potential performance enhancers for athletes, we will discuss other supplements that athletes take. While there are hundreds or even thousands of additional supplements, we will focus on a few of the most popular: multivitamins, iron, vitamin D and calcium, curcumin and turmeric, and collagen, plus several sleep and recovery aids.

Multivitamins

The 2018 Consumer Survey on Dietary Supplements reported that 70 to 75 percent of U.S. adults over the age of 35 are taking a multivitamin at any given time, and about $30 billion is spent annually on multivitamins.

The consensus from the literature is clear. Despite what you might read or hear, it is unnecessary for most athletes to take a multivitamin as long as they follow a well-balanced overall diet and consume adequate total calories regularly (Williams 2004). When elite athletes training at the Australian Institute of Sport were supplemented with a multivitamin for seven to eight months during training, no performance effects were seen (Williams 2004). While it is likely safe for most athletes to take up to 100 percent of the recommended dietary allowance (RDA) for most vitamins, it is not likely to enhance performance, only to save money. My advice is to instead focus on eating a wide variety of foods and taking in adequate total energy (calories) to fuel your athletic life.

Iron

Adequate iron intake and status is often measured in athletes and nonathletes. Iron is a key mineral required throughout the body for many metabolic functions as well as energy production (Latunde-Dada 2012). Suboptimal iron status can result from many factors including inadequate intake of dietary iron; poor availability of the iron that is consumed; inadequate total energy intake; menstrual and other blood loss; high-altitude training; excessive iron losses in sweat, urine, or feces; and foot-strike hemolysis (Maughan et al. 2018).

Altitude training, popular among endurance athletes, requires the body to increase red blood cell production (albeit with higher iron requirements), while exertional exercise increases red blood cell production and thus the need for iron (Kaufman 2018). Iron deficiency is caused by decreased red blood cell production due to low iron availability. Symptoms appear once this low iron availability has progressed to true iron deficiency and include fatigue, pale skin, weakness, dizziness, headaches, decreased aerobic capacity, and overall decreased physical ability (Kaufman 2018). Athletes who fail to meet their nutritional needs and are training in a state of low energy availability (see chapter 10 for more on under-fueling and disordered eating in athletes) often experience changes in sex hormones and menstrual dysfunction (in women) as well as low iron status.

Athletes should have their serum iron measured by a doctor and should also monitor serum ferritin, transferrin saturation, zinc protoporphyrin, hemoglobin, hematocrit, and mean corpuscular volume to help determine the severity and stage of iron deficiency (Gibson 2005). Following these lab tests, athletes may require supplementation with iron at or above the RDA of 18 milligrams per day for women and 8 milligrams per day for men, and would also benefit from including more iron-rich foods in their diet and cooking in a cast-iron skillet. Iron can be found in both plant and animal food sources. (See table 8.2.) Also note that plant sources of iron should be paired with another food that is high in vitamin C to increase absorption (Kaufman 2018).

Athletes who have an iron deficiency should consult a registered sports dietitian, who can help assess their total energy needs as well as counsel them on iron-rich foods and ways to optimize iron absorption. Athletes should also be followed by their medical doctor, who can perform repeat blood tests to determine when it is appropriate to decrease and possibly

TABLE 8.2   Iron-Rich Foods From Plant and Animal Sources

Animal sources	Iron content (mg)	Plant sources	Iron content (mg)
Oysters, 3 oz	8 mg	Fortified cereals, one serving	6.9 mg (fortified oat), up to 18 mg for fortified dry cereals
Liver, 3 oz	5 mg	Lentils, 1/2 cup	3 mg
Sardines, 3 oz	2 mg	Kidney beans, 1/2 cup	2 mg
Lean beef, 3 oz	2 mg	Chickpeas, 1/2 cup	2 mg
Eggs, two whole	2 mg	Pumpkin seeds, 1 oz	0.9 mg
Tuna, 3 oz	1 mg	Enriched whole grain bread, one slice	1 mg
Chicken, 3 oz	1 mg	Molasses, 1 tbsp	0.9 mg
Turkey, 3 oz	1 mg	Tofu, 3 oz	3 mg
		Baked potato, 3 oz	2 mg
		White beans, 1/2 cup	4 mg
		Cashew nuts, 1 oz (18 nuts)	2 mg
		Peanut butter, 2 tbsp	0.6 mg
		Dark green vegetables, cooked, 1/2 cup	3 mg (spinach)

Data from U.S. Department of Agriculture, *FoodData Central* (2019). http://fdc.nal.usda.gov.

cease iron supplementation. Athletes should not supplement without first knowing they are iron deficient, because excess iron intake can lead to iron overload. Iron overload is a condition categorized by increased oxidative damage as well as polythemia, increased blood viscosity, and increased risk of cardiovascular problems, especially when compounded by exertion or extreme heat (Kaufman 2018).

Calcium and Vitamin D

Many athletes are aware of their need to take in adequate calcium and vitamin D but are unsure of when or how much to take. The most important first step for bone and overall health as well as performance of any athlete is to ensure adequate total intake of energy, protein, fat, and carbohydrate as well as vitamins, minerals, and fluids in order to support increased training demands (Kunstel 2005). Compared to most sedentary individuals, athletes have higher needs for energy and for many vitamins and minerals due to both increased stress on the body with exertion and increased losses via the gastrointestinal tract, sweat, urine, and feces. Regarding calcium specifically, the National Institute of Health (NIH), National Academy of Science (NAS), and U.S. Department of Agriculture (USDA) all set requirements based on the goal of preventing osteoporosis.

Calcium is not only needed for bone health, but is also crucial for muscle contraction, nerve impulse conduction, blood pressure and heartbeat regulation, water balance, immune function, and energy and fat metabolism (Kunstel 2005). Although calcium intake is extremely important from childhood through the late 20s, when peak bone mass is generally reached (Kunstel 2005), our need for calcium does not stop there. Throughout our lives, our bones are being continually resorbed or broken down and then created anew, so our need for calcium and vitamin D remain. After menopause, most women will lose 2 to 3 percent of their bone mineral density within 5 to 10 years, and the U.S. Center for Disease Control (CDC) reports that 25 percent of women older than 65 and 5 percent of men older than 65 have osteoporosis (CDC 2019).

Weight-bearing exercise has been shown to help increase bone mineral density throughout adulthood. Swimming and other low- or nonimpact sports, however, have a negative effect on bone mineral density, so those athletes should also incorporate weight-bearing exercise into their regular fitness and health routine. Finally, there is a high risk of low bone mineral density and bone fracture in athletes with low energy availability (those who fail to take in adequate total energy and total protein to meet their daily needs), especially for female athletes with menstrual dysfunction (Kunstel 2005).

See table 8.3 to help you quickly identify your calcium needs.

Many calcium salts have been studied, and the highest absorption rates have been found when calcium carbonate (which should be taken with food) or calcium citrate (which can be taken with or without food) are taken. The NIH states that 43 percent of all U.S. adults take a supplement that contains calcium, while 70 percent of older women do so. They also explain that calcium absorption rates are low: only about 30 percent of calcium from food is absorbed, and this declines by 15 to 20 percent for postmenopausal women and all adults after age 70. If you do require a supplement of more than 500 milligrams, calcium should be taken in split doses and spread throughout (Kunstel 2005). I caution you against taking bone meal sources of calcium, because they have been known to contain lead and cadmium, which can be toxic. Since there is no laboratory test for calcium, we cannot gauge an athlete's needs based on measurable criteria in regular blood testing and need to rely on other information including total nutritional intake, bone density, menstrual function history, and bone mineral density.

Adequate calcium intake can be obtained from foods as well. For most people, 70 percent of our calcium intake comes from milk and dairy products including cheese and yogurt (Kunstel 2005). Those who avoid dairy or need additional calcium-rich foods should look to kale, turnip greens, broccoli, tofu, and calcium-fortified juices and foods to obtain adequate dietary calcium. See table 8.4 for good food sources of calcium.

TABLE 8.3 Calcium Needs by Age

Calcium needs	Age or group
1,000 mg/day	Women ages 25-50 years
1,500 mg/day	Postmenopausal women not on estrogen replacement therapy
1,500-2,000 mg/day	Women with amenorrhea or athletes with low energy availability
1,200 mg/day	All adults over 50 years

Data from National Institutes of Health, Office of Dietary Supplements (2019).

TABLE 8.4 Calcium Content of Foods

Dairy foods	Calcium (mg)	Nondairy sources	Calcium (mg)
Skim or low-fat milk, 1 cup	300	Sardines with bones, 3 oz	325
Whole milk, 1 cup	276	Soy milk, 1 cup	300
Yogurt, 8 oz	300-415	Fortified orange juice, 8 oz	300-350
American cheese, 1 oz	200	Tofu, 1/2 cup raw, firm	250
Mozzarella cheese, 1 oz	200	Fortified cereal, 1 serving	150
Cottage cheese, 1/2 cup	70	Beans, cooked, 1 cup	80-140
		Chia seeds, 1 tbsp	76
		Broccoli, cooked, 1/2 cup	~20
		Kale, cooked, 1/2 cup	~45

The balance of calcium in our bodies is further complicated by several factors. While adequate protein is necessary for optimal bone health, excessive protein intake, specifically from animal sources, may lead to increased urinary loss of calcium from our bodies. The same goes for excessive sodium, caffeine, and alcohol intake, all of which are common in our society and even among athletes. More research is needed in this area, however, to further clarify the relationships between foods and beverages we ingest and calcium absorption and status; recent studies have found that while it is true that excessive protein intake increases calcium excretion, that may also trigger an increase in calcium absorption as well, leading to a net neutral effect.

Phosphorous and caffeine intake may also affect our bones. Some phosphorous is needed to enhance calcium uptake into bones, but excessive intake may lead to decreased bone metabolism. Consumption of carbonated beverages has been linked to lower bone density, possibly because of a combination of less calcium intake (from replacing milk with soda) and an increase in phosphate and caffeine intake leading to increased calcium excretion from our bodies (NIH 2019). Additionally, phytates (found in foods such as wheat bran) and oxalates (found in foods including spinach, sweet potatoes, tea, and walnuts) can also bind to calcium, leading to decreased absorption (Kunstel 2005).

Potassium-rich foods (e.g., legumes, whole grains, fruits, and most vegetables) decrease urinary excretion of calcium. Overall increased produce intake has been linked to decreased calcium excretion. The bottom line here is that eating a balanced and widely varied diet, adequate in total energy, protein, carbohydrate, and fat, rather than focusing on eating a few "superfoods," helps to neutralize each of the issues regarding calcium absorption and generally leads to your healthiest self overall.

One final aspect related to calcium status and bone health is vitamin D. Vitamin D is an essential fat-soluble vitamin that our bodies can make when exposed to adequate sunlight. However, most people I see in my practice, as well as most U.S. adults (especially older adults), have low or inadequate vitamin D status (Kunstel 2005). This is especially problematic for athletes, because adequate vitamin D is important for anyone engaging in strenuous exercise. Furthermore, athletes with low vitamin D levels have been shown to be 3.6 times more likely to develop a stress fracture (Maughan et al. 2018). Luckily, this risk has been shown to decrease by 20 percent when supplementation is taken at 800 IU per day along with 2,000 mg of calcium. Since vitamin D status can be tested by routine bloodwork, it's important for all athletes to have their laboratory markers checked once or twice per year to be able to prevent or quickly treat deficiencies. As with most things, more is not better, so supplementation should be based on laboratory results and monitored after several months of supplementation.

Curcumin and Turmeric

Curcumin is a polyphenol, a chemical compound found in the spice turmeric. Curcumin has been shown to decrease inflammation, pain, and muscle soreness. Early research shows that curcumin might have promising properties such as antibacterial, anti-inflammatory, hypoglycemic, and antioxidant, and that it might serve as a wound-healing or antimicrobial agent. However, it has a low bioavailability and rapid elimination from the body, which has limited its clinical research findings.

Turmeric is a medicinal spice obtained from the root of a plant that is a member of the ginger family. Turmeric has been used in the cuisine and beverages of Asian countries for centuries and has been shown to have anti-inflammatory effects when used in cooking and when taken as a supplement at 5 grams per day (Maughan et al. 2018). Its bioavailability has been shown to increase 2,000 percent when taken with black pepper (Hewlings and Kalman 2017).

Studies have demonstrated decreased oxidative stress and inflammation, decreased muscle soreness and recovery time leading to a subsequent increase in performance, increased performance in working memory, improved mood, and even decreased LDL cholesterol in those taking curcumin (Hewlings and Kalman 2017). Good results have been demonstrated in male cyclists when given 50 milligrams of turmeric (equivalent to 10 mg curcumin) daily for 12 weeks, in 50- to 84-year-old healthy adults when given 400 milligrams of curcumin, and in elite rugby players when given 2 grams of curcumin (Hewlings and Kalman 2017). Overall, scientists and athletes are hopeful that turmeric may help decrease muscle soreness and improve athletic performance over time, but more research is needed.

Curcuminoids have been approved by the FDA as "generally recognized as safe" (GRAS) (Hewlings and Kalman 2017). Hewlings and Kalman also note that studies done in curcumin supplementation seems to indicate its safety. The Joint United Nations and World Health Organization Expert Committee on Food Additives (JECFA) and European Food Safety Authority (EFSA) have set the allowable daily intake (ADI) value of curcumin at 0 to 3 milligrams per kilogram (0-1 mg/lb) of body weight.

Curcumin should not be taken by those who have gallbladder problems or bleeding disorders or who take a blood-thinning medication. Supplementation with turmeric should be ceased at least two weeks prior to any scheduled surgery because it may slow blood clotting. Diabetics should take caution because curcumin might also lower blood sugar.

Collagen

Supplements containing collagen are often touted as having the effects of decreasing joint pain, increasing muscle mass, and supporting connective tissue. Supplementing with collagen or gelatin has been studied at 5 to 15 grams per day or 10 grams of collagen hydrolysate along with 50 milligrams of vitamin C and has shown promising results. It has been theorized that ingesting collagen will help increase the body's natural collagen production, therefore helping to thicken the cartilage (Maughan et al. 2018).

One study reported increased anabolic effect (growth) in cartilage tissue and decreased joint pain in athletes who supplemented with 10 grams of collagen hydrolysate daily for 24 weeks (Clark et al. 2008). While this sounds promising, more studies are needed to fully understand the mechanism and actual benefits. The good news is that although the benefits of taking collagen are not yet fully understood, collagen supplementation seems to be low risk (Maughan et al. 2018).

Supplementing for a Good Night's Sleep

Most athletes have experienced periods of disturbed or reduced sleep duration or quality while heavily training, busy and stressed, or trying to raise small children. Sleep disturbance is an early sign of overtraining. Insomnia and sleep disturbances are also common among high-level and elite athletes. Sleep issues may be due to many factors including high-intensity training as well as travel to competitions, overall stress and tension, and menopause.

A study from the Australian Institute of Sport by Halson (2014), showed that both athletes and coaches ranked sleep as the most predominant problem related to fatigue and tiredness. The study explained that decreased sleep leads to worsened performance and increased levels of confusion scores and tension, and that 24 hours of sleep deprivation has been shown to lead to depressed mood, increased confusion, decreased running performance, increased RPE, decreased sprint times in team sports, and decreased endurance running performance. The researchers found that even 2.5 hours of restricted sleep for four nights in swimmers led to mood changes, increased depression, tension, fatigue, anger, and decreased muscle strength.

On the flip side, sleep extension, defined as instructing athletes to sleep as much as possible for more than two weeks, led to improved mood, decreased fatigue, faster sprint time, improved throw accuracy in baseball players, and increased sprint time and reaction time in swimmers (Halson 2014). Even taking a 30-minute noontime nap has been shown to increase alertness and athletic performance (Halson 2014). It's clear that athletes should prioritize adequate sleep for both overall daily functioning and athletic performance.

To clarify the term *adequate sleep*, the National Sleep Foundation states that sufficient sleep of seven to nine hours per night is needed for most adults to have an increased quality of life as well as to decrease risk of morbidity and mortality (Taylor et al. 2016). Lack of sleep is estimated to cost billions of dollars annually worldwide in decreased productivity, increased health care costs, and increased number of accidents. Inadequate sleep also contributes to increased incidence of obesity and diabetes, higher circulating levels of the hormones cortisol (the so-called stress hormone) and ghrelin (which serves to increase appetite), and depressed levels of leptin (which help to decrease appetite and food intake) (Halson 2014).

While sufficient sleep helps decrease rates of injury and illness and also promotes maximum performance in subsequent training sessions and competition (Taylor et al. 2016), inadequate sleep has been linked to decreased cognitive function, which is crucial in both skill-based and team sports, impaired learning and memory, impaired immune response, and increased inflammatory markers (Halson 2014). Chronic partial sleep deprivation also leads to alterations in glucose metabolism, appetite, food intake, and even protein synthesis. Studies have shown that getting fewer than six hours of sleep a night for only four nights is sufficient to induce both cognitive and metabolic changes (Halson 2014).

Prescription Sleep Medications

Due to the far-reaching consequences of inadequate sleep on daytime wakefulness and performance, the use of sleep aid medications by both recreational and elite athletes has been on the rise (Taylor et al. 2016). However, many sleep aids have been shown to lead to decreased alertness and reaction time, poorer short-term memory recall, and a general "hangover" feeling, but they have no proven benefits to sleep duration or quality (Taylor et al. 2016). Additionally, dependency can develop in a matter of weeks, and Masters athletes are at higher risk because these medications may lead to accidental overdose, unwanted drug interactions, or accidents due to decreased general alertness (Taylor et al. 2016).

Eating Well, Sleeping Well

Inadequate total nutrition and food intake has been shown to impair sleep function in both athletes and nonathletes. Poor sleep quality is a clinical marker that accompanies eating disorders and low energy availability (Cinosi et al. 2011), is seen across the board in low energy states, and leads to altered leptin levels due to low body fat percentage and semi-starvation. Fasting hormone levels increase as weight is restored and food intake is once again adequate.

In a similar vein, recent studies have shown that those fasting during the celebration of Ramadan exhibit about 1.1 hour per day decrease in total sleep time and a delay in falling asleep of about 1.3 hour versus baseline (Taylor et al. 2016). Numerous studies on inadequate energy availability and eating disorders demonstrate higher incidence of sleep apnea, insomnia, and impaired daytime function in individuals with eating disorders (Tromp et al. 2016).

If you are concerned about getting adequate sleep to help your body repair and recover, you must ensure that you are meeting your overall energy and nutritional intake needs. (See chapter 10.) We will now explore a few popular supplements often taken in an effort to improve sleep duration and quality.

Melatonin

Melatonin is a hormone produced by the pineal gland in the brain that is known to influence sleep. The marketing for melatonin as a sleep aid is prolific. This is mainly based on the fact that increased natural production of melatonin in our bodies in the evening leads to increased synthesis of serotonin, decreased central nervous system stimulation, and increased sleepiness (López-Flores et al. 2018). However, studies on melatonin ingestion before bed are inconclusive at best. Many athletes report unwanted side effects including grogginess, headaches, and daytime sleepiness the next morning. Based on these reported side effects and the unknown long-term safety of taking melatonin, I recommend trying something else instead if you need a better night's sleep.

The only exception to this recommendation might be immediately following long-distance and time-changing travel. Case studies have suggested that taking 3 grams of melatonin 30 minutes before bed combined with outdoor exercise (providing light exposure) during the window of eight to eleven o'clock in the morning and one to four o'clock in the afternoon may help resynchronize sleep faster and reduce jet lag (López-Flores et al. 2018).

L-Tryptophan and Sleep

L-tryptophan is an essential amino acid (EAA), meaning that we must ingest it because our bodies need it but cannot synthesize it on its own. This EAA is found in the lowest concentrations among all amino acids and is critical to both protein synthesis and serotonin production. Increasing the amount of the EAA tryptophan in our bodies is a known way to increase our melatonin and thus may facilitate sleep.

Nutritional interventions for increasing tryptophan and promoting sleep have been a topic of interest for a while now. Studies have shown that taking 1 gram of tryptophan before bed may decrease time to fall asleep and decrease waking time throughout the night (Attele, Xie, and Yuan 2000). As many have experienced, eating foods rich in tryptophan—turkey, milk, oats, bananas, tuna fish, wheat bread, peanuts, or even chocolate—may lead to improved overall sleep quality without any added risk.

Diet Composition and Sleep

Ingesting high glycemic index carbohydrate (white rice, pasta, potato, bread) at least one hour prior to going to bed might promote shorter time to fall asleep. Eating a higher-carb meal before bedtime increases postprandial (postmeal) insulin response as well as tryptophan response, which leads to increased tryptophan available to enter the brain and subsequent increased serotonin production, which promotes sleep.

Adequate overall dietary protein intake has also been shown to facilitate sounder sleep (Halson 2014). Conversely, diets high in fat have been shown to have adverse consequences on sleep duration, especially in postmenopausal women (Halson 2014).

Liquid meals have been shown to lead to increased sleep latency (longer time to fall asleep) versus solid meals. Most importantly, keep in mind that diets inadequate in overall calories have been shown to impact sleep negatively, so make sure that you do eat dinner after tiring evening workouts or long days at the office.

Over the years, many studies have confirmed what you may have been told when you were growing up, that a warm glass of milk or other foods high in tryptophan (including turkey or pumpkin seeds) before bed might help you sleep better. Combining some of these foods, while also ensuring that you consume adequate total protein and carbohydrate, may be your best bet for a good night's sleep.

Tart Cherry Juice

Tart cherry juice is another well-researched supplement that has become popular in the athletic world over the past 10 years. Early studies demonstrated that eating 45 cherries daily led to decreased inflammatory markers in healthy individuals (Kuehl et al. 2010). However, since that is an unrealistic amount of cherries to eat daily, studies turned to tart cherry juice. Many studies have shown potential for this fruit juice to decrease muscle pain and damage after exercise because it is an antioxidant and an anti-inflammatory agent (Kuehl et al. 2010).

Many studies have shown that taking tart cherry juice might aid recovery. One study gave tart cherry juice to both men and women (average age 35.8 years) twice daily for seven days, before and on the day of their Hood to Coast Relay race in Oregon (Kuehl et al. 2010). This is a very hilly, 12-runner team relay event during which each runner completes three segments over 24 hours, totaling 15 to 19 miles per runner. Runners in the tart cherry supplementation group reported decreased pain and high satisfaction with the supplement. Other studies showed that supplementation with tart cherry juice for five days prior to and 48 hours after running a marathon led to faster recovery of muscle strength and reduced inflammation (Kuehl et al. 2010). Many studies have repeated these results in distance runners and other athletes in sports that involve eccentric contraction activities. Vitale, Hueglin, and Broad (2017) reported in their review article that marathoners given 8 ounces of tart cherry juice twice daily for five days prior to and two days after the London Marathon demonstrated decreased inflammatory markers and were able to recover faster. They also found that Olympic athletes given tart cherry juice reported decreased muscle soreness and improved sleep.

To date, the exact mechanism for these benefits is unknown. Improvements may have resulted from both the antioxidant component of tart cherry juice as well as increased carbohydrate intake with juice supplementation (Vitale, Hueglin, and Broad 2017). More sport-specific research is needed, but recent studies show enhanced recovery when athletes were given 250 to 350 milliliters (9-12 oz) of tart cherry juice (or 30 mL [1 oz] of concentrate) twice daily for four to five days prior to and two to three days after the event (Maughan et al. 2018). As with other supplements, if you choose to try this, test it out in a low-key race or competition first to ensure your gastrointestinal tract handles it well.

While it may be worth taking when you are in peak condition and want to recover quickly between one competition and the next (e.g., in a multiple-day stage race; weekend of many games; or prelims, semi-finals, and finals), tart cherry juice should not be taken during training adaptation phases (base and build), because it may only serve to blunt desired training adaptations.

Regarding sleep, some studies have shown that drinking 1 ounce (28 mL) of tart cherry juice concentrate before bed may increase sleep-enhancing melatonin and improve subjective insomnia symptoms when compared to a placebo. Because inflammation can lead to disrupted sleep, taking tart cherry juice, which contains antioxidants and anti-inflammatory phytochemicals, might positively impact sleep. This is important to athletes who experience a high inflammatory load due to heavy training and who are seeking to improve the quality and duration of sleep. In a study of 15 adults older than 65, a twice-daily ingestion of tart cherry juice (reconstituted into 8 ounces both morning and one or two hours before bedtime) for two weeks was associated with statistically significant reductions in insomnia as measured by sleep onset, total sleep time, and sleep efficiency.

L-Theanine

L-theanine is an amino acid naturally present in tea and is another possible and low-risk sleep and recovery aid I use with my athlete clients. L-theanine is known to help promote a feeling of calm. Recent research shows that rowers given 150 milligrams of L-theanine twice daily for six weeks were shown to have significant improvements in post–strenuous exercise immunity (Juszkiewicz et al. 2019), which could have implications for reducing incidence of upper respiratory infections following competition.

A typical cup of tea contains 7.9 to 24 milligrams of L-theanine. At the very least, drinking a warm mug of noncaffeinated tea before bedtime is a great ritual in terms of overall sleep hygiene and might help promote sleep due to its L-theanine content.

Valerian Root

Valerian root is an herbal sleep remedy that has been used by traditional herbalists for years. It can be taken in tea or capsule form and has also shown some promise in terms of helping people fall asleep faster and improve over-all quality of sleep. Several studies have shown that when volunteers were given 400 to 900 milligrams of valerian extract before bed, they reported better sleep quality (versus those taking a placebo) or shorter duration of time to fall asleep (Halson 2014). Halson (2014) also stated that while a few studies showed some positive effect after even a single dose, many studies demonstrated maximal effects after a two-week continual trial. Valerian is classified as GRAS by the U.S. FDA, although there are some reported side effects including drowsiness and dizziness. Studies are needed to determine long-term safety.

Sleep is extremely important for the overall health of all beings, specifically for recovery, immunity, and subsequent performance in athletes. Depending on your specific situation and needs, you can improve your sleep in many ways. See the sidebar for a summary.

Dos and Don'ts of a Better Night's Sleep

Sleep Helpers

- Taking tart cherry juice concentrate one or two hours before bed may help you fall asleep faster.
- Eating a diet with adequate but not excessive protein can improve sleep quality.
- Ingesting high glycemic index carbohydrate one to four hours prior to bedtime can shorten duration to fall asleep.
- Taking 400 milligrams of valerian root extract daily for two weeks may improve sleep quality.
- Eating foods high in L-tryptophan (turkey, pumpkin seeds, milk) or taking 1 gram per day can improve sleep quality.
- Drinking teas that contain L-theanine prior to bedtime can promote a feeling of calm and enhance sleep.

Sleep Destroyers

- Eating a high-fat diet may reduce sleep.
- Not ingesting adequate total energy (calories) may reduce sleep quality and duration.
- Having a liquid instead of solid meal before bed may worsen sleep.

Overall, athletes and the general population are willing to spend billions of dollars annually in hopes of improving their energy, longevity, and performance. While studies show promising benefits of some supplementation in athletes, the onus is on you, the athlete, to do your research, verify that studies prove performance effects, and confirm that what you take is free of contamination or unwanted additives. It is certainly not an easy world to navigate. My professional recommendation is to start by ensuring you are meeting your total energy, carbohydrate, protein, and fat needs, both throughout your day and before, during, and after training, and that you are eating a wide variety of colorful foods from all food groups. Next, it would be wise to have a medical doctor check your bloodwork once or twice a year to identify any possible deficiencies. Thereafter, weigh the potential benefits of any performance-enhancing supplements for you and your specific sport and duration of activity against any possible side effects.

In chapter 9, we will turn our attention to hydration, covering fluid and electrolyte needs for athletes.

9 | Fluid Needs

Maintaining your hydration status is of utmost importance to both your overall health and athletic performance. The first scientific studies demonstrating the importance of maintaining fluid balance in the heat during activity were done by the military. These studies showed that fluid replacement sustained military endurance performance both in the laboratory and in field trials (Sawka, Cheuvront, and Kenefick 2015). Subsequent studies have consistently confirmed the link between hydration status and athletic performance in activities ranging from submaximal exercise to maximal-intensity aerobic performance in both warm and hot environments. Evidence shows that the human thirst response generally results in balanced rehydration following slight dehydration over the course of many hours. However, it has repeatedly been shown that during periods of strenuous physical exercise with high sweat rates, athletes repeatedly underconsume fluids when attempting to maintain their hydration status by simply listening to their thirst (Sawka, Cheuvront, and Kenefick 2015). Baker and Jeukendrup (2014) found that when athletes engage in exercise for more than two hours in one day, the fluid regulatory system is strained such that thirst is often no longer a reliable indicator of fluid needs.

The abundance of available evidence does not support any degree of deliberate dehydration by an athlete in an attempt to improve performance (Maughan and Shirreffs 2010), because substantial and meaningful performance affects may be far-reaching and also well below that which can or have been measured by laboratory studies. Despite these early and thereafter repeated findings confirming the link between maintaining hydration status and sustaining performance in athletes, debate continues over this surprisingly controversial topic (Sawka, Cheuvront, and Kenefick 2015). Let's dive in further to find out the truth about the athlete's daily fluid and sodium needs.

Water: It's What We Are Made Of!

The human body is said to be made up of about 60 percent water, although it is important to note that trained athletes often have a higher total body water content due to a higher percentage of lean body mass (LBM), which is comprised of 70 to 80 percent water versus fat mass (FM), which is only about 10 percent water. Therefore, as an athlete, your body may fall in the range of 60 to 75 percent water (ACSM et al. 2007). Wherever you fall on the fluid scale, one thing is certain: water is an important aspect of your body to maintain.

Sweating is the body's automatic response to a need to dissipate heat as the body temperature rises above what is optimal. Sweat rate is quite variable both within individuals (due to differences in environmental temperature and humidity, air motion, clothing and equipment, body weight, heat acclimatization, and intensity of exercise) and between individuals (due to differences in genetics and metabolic efficiency) (ACSM et al. 2007).

You may be wondering just how much water you should you be drinking each day. According to the Institute of Medicine of the National Academies Dietary Reference Intakes (DRI) Consensus Report from 2005, the general recommendations for "healthy sedentary people in temperate climates" are 2.7 liters (92 oz) of fluid from all beverages and foods for women and 3.7 liters (126 oz) of fluid from all beverages and foods for men (Institute of Medicine 2005). However, translating this for athletes is difficult, because athletes are working in a wide range of different environmental conditions, at various intensities and states of heat acclimatization, and for a wide range of hours each day, which leads to daily fluid needs that can range from 1 liter (34 oz) per day to up to 10 liters (340 oz) per day (Baker and Jeukendrup 2014).

On average, about 80 percent of your total water intake comes from drinking water and other beverages, while about 20 percent comes from the foods you eat. However, some foods (e.g., watermelon, strawberries, cucumbers) contain more than 90 percent water, while others (e.g., crackers, oils, sugars, chips, seeds) contain very little. See table 9.1 for a list of high– and low–water content foods.

TABLE 9.1   High–Water Content and Low–Water Content Foods

Foods with greater than 90% water content	Foods with less than 20% water content
Watermelon	Butters and oils
Strawberries	Sugar and candies
Grapefruit	Cookies and crackers
Cantaloupe	Nuts and seeds
Broccoli	Avocado
Cucumber and zucchini	Chips
Lettuce and cabbage	Dry cereals

Busting Hydration Myths

Let's clear up some confusion about hydrating fluids right off the bat. Not only plain water, but also seltzers, milk, juices, and even caffeinated beverages including tea and coffee count toward your daily fluid intake goal. You have undoubtedly heard that caffeine is a diuretic and will cause you to lose more water than you drink, but this has been disproven. Evidence clearly shows that any diuretic effect of caffeine is transient and generally does not lead to decreased total body water.

Additionally, you may have heard (correctly) that as an athlete, you require additional total daily fluid if you are eating a diet very high in protein. However, those increased fluid needs are likely negligible unless your protein intake is extremely excessive. (If that is the case, see chapters 5 through 7 on carbohydrate, protein, and healthy fat.) Sawka (1992) found that for every 100 grams of protein intake, we require 700 milliliters (about 25 oz) of fluid (Guyton and Hall 2000). Since the overall fluid needs of an athlete generally lie in the range of more than 3 or 4 liters (106-141 oz) a day, an additional few grams of protein should not affect your overall hydration needs significantly. If, however, you feel that you are following an excessively high protein diet, I recommend that you consult with a board-certified sports dietitian (RDN, CSSD) to ensure you are both meeting your fluid needs and not exceeding safe intake for protein or missing out on carbohydrate or fat in its place.

Hydration: A Moving Target for Masters Athletes

The Institute of Medicine (IOM) report says that those who are very physically active or live in hot climates may need to consume more water than they recommend for the general population. This makes sense, since sweat rate increases with training and racing, which in turn greatly increases total daily fluid intake needs.

For the general population, it has been shown that transient decreases in hydration status due to underconsumption of total fluids, exposure to increased heat, gastrointestinal losses, or increases in respiration will return to normal hydration over the next 12 to 24 hours by the kidneys adjusting urine output appropriately and by following one's thirst (ACSM et al. 2007). However, athletes, especially those who engage in long or strenuous sessions regularly or complete more than one session on any given day, should pay extra attention to ensure they are keeping up with their fluid intake needs. The Academy of Nutrition and Dietetics and American College of Sports Medicine Joint Position Statement of Nutrition and Athletic Performance (Thomas, Erdman, and Burke 2016) explains that our bodies generate heat when muscles are contracted, which leads to an increased sweat rate in order to maintain a safe body temperature. The statement warns athletes

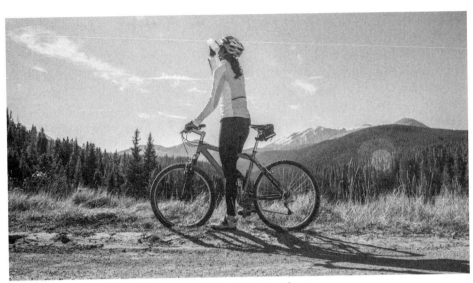

Age, exercise intensity, and climate affect fluid needs.

Jacobs Stock Photography Ltd/DigitalVision/Getty Images

that if we do not increase our fluid and sodium intake to match these needs, we experience hypovolemia (decreased plasma or blood volume), which may lead to cardiac strain, increased body temperature, increased glycogen utilization, and altered central nervous system (CNS) function. Therefore, we should maintain euhydration (a normal state of body water content) to prevent these adverse effects. Although the kidneys do their best to decrease urine output in response to exercise, we also want to choose drinks that contain both sodium and flavor to increase our drive to drink voluntarily.

Another complicating factor is that the sweat rate of an athlete can range widely from 0.3 to 2.4 liters (10.6-84.5 oz) per hour. Changes in sweat rate occur based on intensity and duration of exercise or competition, fitness, heat and humidity, altitude, and an athlete's state of heat acclimatization (Thomas, Erdman, and Burke, 2016). The range of sodium content in each liter of sweat also varies tremendously from athlete to athlete and also within an athlete's year or season as the athlete acclimates to warmer weather and increases sweat output. The fact that a liter of sweat may contain 300 to 2,400 milligrams of sodium and that athletes may be losing a liter of sweat per hour makes it quite challenging to know just how much fluid to take in.

Masters athletes have additional variables to consider. For starters, older athletes have less total body water than younger athletes. Infants start at about 80 percent water. Water content decreases as we age, dropping to 60 to 70 percent. Furthermore, our ability to concentrate urine in our kidneys declines, because our number of functioning nephrons diminishes as the decades pass. This is further compounded by the fact that our kidneys are already decreasing urine production during exercise in order to conserve water to account for fluid losses from sweat. We begin to experience a blunted thirst response as well, meaning that our ability to detect when we are thirsty also declines with age (ACSM et al. 2007), further increasing our risk of dehydration during exercise.

Other confounding factors include decreased overall sweat rate as we age (Balmain et al. 2018) as well as medications we may take to control other medical issues that develop with age. Walter and Lenz (2011) caution against the use of NSAIDS (nonsteroidal anti-inflammatory drugs) such as ibuprofen, a class of medication many athletes use regularly to decrease pain after training or injury and to prevent pain during training or competitions. This practice is discouraged because such mediations have not been shown to prevent muscle soreness and have been shown to decrease glomerular filtration rate (GFR) or kidney function, which can contribute to increased risk of kidney damage when an athlete is or becomes dehydrated. Additionally, as we age, it will take us longer to restore fluid balance once we do become dehydrated (ACSM et al. 2007) because of both the aforementioned decreased thirst response and age-related increased resting plasma osmolality (the body's electrolyte-water balance).

Sweat rates vary so widely that general recommendations for total fluid and sodium intake per hour simply do not work. Therefore, I highly recommend that you conduct sweat testing periodically during training so that you are aware of how much you sweat per hour and how much you need to drink. See figure 9.1 for a sweat test worksheet you can complete each season or as needed. To accurately assess your individual sweat rate, you should perform this test multiple times in each sport and each climate or season in which you train and compete. Body weight measurements before and after exercise should ideally be taken nude or in as little dry clothing so that sweat absorbed into clothing after exercise is not weighed. Additionally, since you might not be willing or able to collect your urine to determine the volume of fluid lost there, you should conduct your sweat tests on workouts that are long enough for you to sweat but not long enough for you to need to urinate. Most people find that 60- to 90-minute workouts work well.

Water, Water Everywhere, but What About Salt?

In addition to taking in adequate total daily fluid, we need to think about our sodium needs and intake. The IOM report states that healthy adults ages 19 to 50 should consume 1.5 grams of sodium and 2.3 grams of chloride (or 3.8 grams of salt) each day to replace losses due to respiration, urine and fecal output, and insensible losses through our skin. The tolerable upper limit (UL), or the maximum amount thought to be safe for consumption for the population at large, is currently 5.8 grams per day. While this amount may sound high to many of you, it has been shown that more than 95 percent of U.S. men and more than 75 percent of U.S. women exceed that amount daily, in large part due to overconsumption of prepared and processed foods. Before you start calculating your average daily sodium intake, note that depending on your activity level and sweat rate these numbers may not apply to you, because you also need to replace additional fluid and sodium for each hour of exercise you engage in daily. The goal for most athletes, as we will discuss shortly, is to match your fluid intake to your sweat loss during exercise to ensure you limit body weight loss due to sweat to less than 2 percent of your body weight.

Sweat Test Worksheet for Athletes

Date: _____   Temperature: _____

Sport: _____   Humidity: _____

Preworkout weight (no clothes, in pounds)	
Duration of workout	
Fluid intake during workout (if any, in ounces)	
Postworkout weight (no clothes, in pounds)	

Please also note whether you think you are a "salty" sweater. You likely fall into this category if you've experienced frequent muscle cramping or if you find yourself covered in a layer of salt upon completion of your workouts.

Once you have conducted several sweat tests, use the following formula to calculate your sweat rate. Keep workouts short enough to avoid having to measure urine volume.

Sweat rate = (pre-exercise weight – postexercise weight) × 16 oz of sweat lost + (fluid consumed – urine volume) / exercise time in hours

Weight is in pounds and fluid is in ounces.

For example: A soccer player weighed 140 pounds before practice and 137 pounds after a two-hour practice. She drank 24 ounces of a sport drink during her workout. She did not urinate during the workout.

Her sweat rate = (140–137 lb) × 16 oz = 48 oz + 24 oz / 2 hours = 36 oz/hour

If this athlete repeated this sweat test several times under similar environmental conditions, she would say that she sweats about 36 ounces per hour and therefore should aim to replace as close to that as possible during practices and games in similar conditions.

FIGURE 9.1 Sweat test worksheet for athletes.

Data from Centers for Disease Control and Prevention (2011). https://www.cdc.gov/nceh/hsb/extreme/Heat_Illness/Sweat%20Rate%20Calculation.pdf

From L. Antonucci, *High-Performance Nutrition for Masters Athletes*. (Champaign, IL: Human Kinetics, 2022).

As we discussed in chapter 3, if you have high blood pressure or hypertension (HTN) or other conditions such as diabetes or kidney disease, you may have been told to consume less than the UL for sodium. About 25 percent of all U.S. adults and over 50 percent of U.S. adults over age 60 have HTN (IOM 2005): U.S. men consume between 7.8 and 11.8 grams per day of sodium while U.S. women consume 2.4 to 2.6 grams per day, and only one in four U.S. adults are active regularly to help sweat out any extra salt they take in. If this applies to you, you may want to limit your overall salt intake to 1.5 to 2.4 grams per day on nonexercise days, then increase your sodium intake to meet your needs during heavy training sessions.

Potassium Is Also Necessary

If you were told you have HTN, you will likely want to increase your intake of potassium-rich foods, because adequate potassium intake can help counterbalance the adverse effects of high sodium intake while also decreasing the risk of kidney stones and preserving bone as we age. In addition to helping lower blood pressure, potassium, which is found in most fruits and vegetables and in some other foods, helps with muscle contraction and to regulate and maintain fluid balance. The caveat is that most Americans consume barely more than half the recommended amount of potassium each day. In fact, the 2015-2020 Dietary Guidelines for Americans listed potassium as both an under consumed nutrient and a nutrient of public health concern. See table 9.2 for a list of potassium-rich foods to ensure you are meeting your needs. The Guidelines recommend that adult males older than 19 years consume 3,400 mg of potassium a day from foods and adult women consume more than 2,600 mg of potassium a day from foods. There is no UL for potassium intake from foods.

Next, we will discuss your increased needs before, during, and after your exercise sessions.

Pre-Exercise Hydration

Since hypohydration (uncompensated loss of body water that is greater than expected normal daily fluctuation) is known to adversely affect performance outcomes, it is important to start each training session and competition in a state of euhydration, which requires adequate food and water intake during the 8 to 12 hours prior to each session. Unfortunately, but not surprisingly, research demonstrates that many athletes begin exercise already dehydrated. To ensure optimal hydration status at the start of each session and to promote voiding prior to the start of training or your completion, you should aim to drink 5 to 10 milliliters per kilogram of body weight (2-4 mL/lb) in the two to four hours prior (Thomas, Erdman, and Burke 2016). Another helpful tool is to monitor your urine color, frequency, and volume to assess your fluid status

TABLE 9.2 Dietary Sources of Potassium

More than 900 mg/serving	400-900 mg/serving	200-400 mg/serving	<200 mg/serving
Grapefruit juice, 1 cup	Winter squash, 1 cup	Banana, orange, one small or medium	Plum, one small
Soybeans, 1/2 cup	Cantaloupe, honeydew, 1 cup, cubed	Peach, nectarine, pear, kiwi, one medium	Grapefruit, half medium
Canned tomato purée, 1 cup	Papaya, mango, 1 cup	Strawberries, mango, blackberries, 1 cup	Cherries, 1/2 cup
Swiss chard, 1 cup, cooked	Tomato or orange juice, 1 cup	Molasses, 1 tbsp	Canned peaches, 1/2 cup
Beets, 1 cup, cooked	Dried fruit (raisins, prunes, apricots, mango), 1/4 cup	Tofu, 1/2 cup	Blueberries, raspberries, 1 cup, raw
Plantain, 1 medium to large	Avocado, 1/2 medium	Peanut butter, 2 tbsp, or peanuts, 1/4 cup	Watermelon, 1 cup
	Potatoes, white or sweet, 1 cup or one medium	Milk, cottage cheese, yogurt, 1 cup	Kale, spinach, lettuce, cucumber, celery, 1 cup, raw
	Tomatoes, 1 cup raw or 1/2 cup, cooked/sauce	Brussels sprouts, carrots, broccoli, 1 cup	Zucchini, okra, cauliflower, eggplant, 1/2 cup, cooked
	Dark leafy greens (spinach, kale, Swiss chard, bok choy, mustard greens, beet greens), 1 cup, cooked	Green beans, peas, corn, beets, asparagus, 1/2 cup, cooked	Applesauce, 1 cup
	Beans (white, baked, lima, soy, pink), 1/2 cup, cooked	Lentils, black, navy, pinto, kidney beans, 1/2 cup, cooked	Apple, one medium, raw

Data from U.S. Department of Agriculture, USDA National Nutrient Database for Standard Reference Legacy (2018).

(Maughan and Shirreffs 2008). Urine should be pale yellow in color when you are well hydrated. Darker color (apple juice color) and low volume urine generally indicate dehydration and may require an additional 3 to 5 milliliters per kilogram of body weight (1-2 mL/lb) of fluid about two hours prior (ACSM et al. 2007). Keep in mind that urine color can be affected by B-complex vitamins—which turns it bright yellow or orange—as well as some foods, medications, and food dyes (Maughan and Shirreffs 2008). Remember that you are looking for overall clues to help you better understand your fluid needs and status, and for changes from your normal. See table 9.3 for guidelines on how to determine your specific pre-exercise hydration needs.

You may also want to include some foods or fluids with sodium to help increase your thirst response, drive to drink, and fluid retention. See the list below for some high-sodium foods to include before or after long, strenuous sweat sessions.

TABLE 9.3 Pre-Exercise Fluid Intake Guidelines

Fluid needs	For 120 lb (54 kg) athlete	For 160 lb (73 kg) athlete	For 200 lb (91 kg) athlete
Drink 5-10 mL/kg (2-4 mL/lb) of body weight during the two to four hours prior to training or competition	256-341 mL (9-12 oz)	341-483 mL (12-17 oz)	426-597 mL (15-21 oz)
Drink an additional 3-5 mL/kg (1-2 mL/lb) of body weight about two hours prior if urine is still dark in color	142-256 mL (5-9 oz)	199-341 mL (7-12 oz)	256-426 mL (9-15 oz)

Dietary Sources of Sodium

- Cured meats including cold cuts
- Soups
- Vegetable/tomato juices
- Pasta sauce
- Condiments including ketchup and BBQ sauce
- Smoked salmon
- Canned foods including beans, vegetables, and seafood (canned tuna)
- Salted popcorn
- Pickled vegetables
- Salted nuts
- Ready-to-eat breakfast cereals
- Cheeses
- Pizza
- Boxed and prepared/convenience foods

In an attempt to preload or hyperhydrate prior to exercise, some athletes have tried using glycerol or other plasma expanders however, this practice has been shown to increase urine output without improved performance. Additionally, they are now banned by the World Anti-Doping Agency (WADA) and are therefore not recommended.

Fluid and Sodium Needs During Exercise

Maintaining hydration status during exercise and competition is one of the most important nutritional strategies for any performance athlete. Doing so will help maintain heart rate, stroke volume, cardiac output, skin blood flow, core body temperature, rating of perceived exertion (RPE), and overall performance. You are probably aware of the health risks associated with heat stress and heat illness due to exercising in extreme heat, but performance will generally suffer as a result of dehydration long before those two dangerous conditions become a concern. In addition, many athletes do not fully comprehend the far-reaching adverse effects of dehydration including exacerbated strain on our cardiovascular system, decreased blood flow to the brain, elevated core temperature, increased skeletal muscle glycogen use, increased fatigue and decreased mood and brain function (Sawka, Cheuvront, and Kenefick 2015). Fluid losses will generally be lower when you are exercising in a cooler environment, as will your body's tolerance for withstanding the state of underhydration (ACSM et al. 2007). However, environmental heat stress increases our body's sweat rate response and fluid losses through our skin to keep our body cool. When exercising in humid environments, our skin is damp, which decreases our initial sweat response, increasing the chances of our bodies overheating. Over time, a training response occurs as we acclimate to training and racing in the heat by producing a higher volume of sweat to keep cool (ACSM et al. 2007).

Upon initial training, introduction to the heat, or anytime an athlete becomes acutely dehydrated, the body increases the sweat concentration of sodium and chloride in order to conserve fluids. However, over time, heat acclimatization occurs, leading to increased total sweat rate and decreased sodium content of sweat by up to 50 percent for any individual athlete (ACSM et al. 2007).

While neither sweat rate nor electrolyte concentration of sweat are predictable by knowing an athlete's gender or age alone, an increase in ambient temperature results in a near-universal impairment in aerobic performance across all athletes (Sawka, Cheuvront, and Kenefick 2015). However, since the extent to which sweat rate and performance deterioration occur varies widely, each athlete's output and needs require individual consideration and investigation. It is generally understood that most athletes' hydration goal should be to customize their fluid replacement plan in order to prevent less than 2 percent loss of body weight due to sweat in order to prevent degradation in performance. Many studies have shown that a decrease of 2 to 7 percent of body mass consistently decreases endurance-training performance in distances beginning with 1,500 meters (Maughan and Shirreffs 2008). Performance deteriorates with dehydration even in temperate conditions but is greatly impaired when more than 2 percent body weight is lost, exercise session is longer than 90 minutes, or temperature exceeds 30°C (86°F). Team sport athletes are not immune to the effects of even low-level dehydration. One study showed that soccer skills test performance decreased by 5 percent in experimental conditions when no drinking was allowed compared to when athletes were allowed to consume fluids during activity (Maughan and Shirreffs 2008). Maughan and Shirreffs (2008) also show that mild dehydration adversely affects mood and cognitive function.

Any loss of body weight exceeding 1 to 2 percent of pre-exercise weight requires further examination and discussion, since for most athletes, and especially for those performing in warm, hot, or high-altitude environments, even this seemingly small loss of body weight due to sweat has been shown to adversely affect performance (Sawka, Cheuvront, and Kenefick 2015). For example, time trial performance has been shown to decrease significantly in both male and female cyclists who were dehydrated to the point of having lost only 1 to 2 percent of their body weight (Logan-Sprenger et al. 2012; Logan-Sprenger et al. 2015). They found that well-trained male cyclists completed a 5-kilometer hill climb faster when dehydration was minimized to 1.4 percent body weight loss compared to 2.2 percent or greater body weight loss. The authors' conclusion is that high-intensity performance cannot be maintained when about 2 to 3 percent dehydration occurs. Possible mechanisms for this include not only the dehydration itself, but also an accompanying increase in muscle glycogen use in dehydrated athletes over the two-hour cycling trial. During their studies, male athletes were found to increase muscle glycogen use by up to 24 percent, while female athletes were found to increase muscle glycogen use by up to 31 percent, which alone can limit performance. The authors also noted increased heart rate by 4 to 9 beats per minute beginning at 20 minutes into the trial and continuing throughout, increased whole-body stress and reported feelings of decreased concentration, headaches, and increased RPE during exercise (Logan-Sprenger et al. 2012).

Maintaining close-to-baseline body weight from before to after training or competition also helps athletes avoid consequences of dehydration. Severe hypohydration is a concern for all athletes, because anytime 6 to 10 percent of body weight is lost due to sweating or fluid losses the athlete is at high risk for decreased cardiac output, decreased sweat production (and thus increased body temperature), decreased blood flow to skin and muscle, decreased performance and function, and increased risk of heat illness and heat stroke (ACSM et al. 2007). See table 9.4 for calculation of dehydration status by body weight.

TABLE 9.4   Fluid and Body Weight Losses by the Numbers

Dehydration status	Resulting weight for 120 lb (54 kg) athlete	Resulting weight for 160 lb (73 kg) athlete	Resulting weight for 200 lb (91 kg) athlete
2% loss of body weight: maximum acceptable fluid loss for most athletes	117.6 lb (53.3 kg) (2.4 lb [1.1 kg] fluid loss)	156.8 lb (71.1 kg) (3.2 lb [1.5 kg] fluid loss)	196 lb (89 kg) (4 lb [2 kg] fluid loss)
3% loss of body weight: possible maximum acceptable fluid loss for anaerobic sports, cold weather, technical skill sports	116 lb (54 kg) (3.6 lb [1.6 kg] fluid loss)	155.2 lb (70.4 kg) (4.8 lb [2.2 kg] fluid loss)	194 lb (88 kg) (6 lb [3 kg] fluid loss)
6% loss of body weight: severe dehydration	112.8 lb (51.2 kg) (7.2 lb [3.3 kg] fluid loss)	150.4 lb (68.2 kg) (9.6 lb [4.4 kg] fluid loss)	188 lb (85 kg) (12 lb [5 kg] fluid loss)

Recent research suggests that athletes engaging in cold environments, in anaerobic sports, or in sports with high technical skill involvement might only need to ensure their hydration status does not dip below a 3 percent decrease in body weight due to sweat loss and dehydration to maintain performance (Thomas, Erdman, and Burke 2016). However, this kind of loss should not occur on a regular basis because of the aforementioned repercussions of training or competing while dehydrated. As we have already discussed, (see Figure 9.2 for sweat rate testing guidelines), each athlete should estimate changes in hydration by monitoring changes in body weight during exercise. (See figure 9.1.) It is well supported (Maughan and Shirreffs 2008) that sweat rates can be estimated when both fluid intake and urine output (if any) are also measured.

If it is necessary to more accurately assess sodium content of sweat, sweat samples from the skin during exercise, ideally multiple times and at multiple sites (forearm, forehead, chest, back, thigh, and calf) can be collected and analyzed. Abnormally high or abnormally low measured sodium concentrations of sweat should be treated with caution and repeated if possible. If that is not possible, athletes can look for salt residue on dark or black clothing left after sweat has evaporated. The more residue, the higher sodium content of sweat. Due to the numerous factors influencing an individual athlete's sweat rate, several measurements should be taken under similar environmental conditions to approximate fluid and sodium needs for that athlete under similar conditions.

Let's turn now to an elite athlete who has had to go to great lengths to understand and meet her hydration needs in order to complete at the highest level.

Hydration Helpers

It is well known that consuming beverages that contain both sodium and flavor increase our drive to drink, which helps athletes achieve optimal performance. Additionally, athletes see benefits when taking in carbohydrate during exercise in an effort to improve performance (Maughan and Shirreffs 2010). As previously discussed, Masters athletes need to pay heightened attention to meeting fluid needs due to age-related decreases in thirst response. This is further compounded for those Masters athletes who are salty sweaters, higher-volume sweaters (sweating at a rate of >1.2 L/hr [42.2 oz/hr]), or who exercise for more than 2 hr/day. These athletes will maintain hydration status better—and therefore feel and perform better—drinking beverages with carbohydrate and sodium than drinking water alone (Thomas, Erdman, and Burke 2016). This additive effect of both adequate fluid and carbohydrate intake has been shown to ring true for both male and female athletes over a wide range of activities in varying environmental conditions (Maughan and Shirreffs 2008).

Cold beverages are generally preferable because they will help decrease body temperature and promote fluid intake in most athletes. Studies consistently show a significantly smaller rise in core body temperature during exercise when athletes consume cold beverages versus room temperature fluids (LaFata et al. 2012). This slower increase in core temp helps athletes to maintain pace and performance for longer, and is advised whenever possible. Freezing water or sport drink bottles until as close as possible just prior to training or competition can help keep fluids cold during longer events, and is a widely utilized strategy.

Your best plan as an athlete is to monitor your weight before and after exercise to prevent excess body weight loss. Most athletes should start by drinking 0.4 to 0.8 liters per hour (14.1-28.2 oz/hr), spreading out that fluid intake out through training and competition sessions (Sawka, Cheuvront, and Kenefick 2015). Special attention should be paid anytime an athlete will be sweating for more than three hours (e.g., triathletes, marathoners, and tennis and soccer players on multiple match or game days), because incidence of both dehydration and hyperhydration increase with longer-duration exercise sessions. Athletes wearing heavy equipment (e.g., football, hockey) may lose up to 8 liters (272 oz) of fluid per day during training, so must pay careful attention to fluid balance between sessions. Those training in dry climates or at high altitudes will have increased respiratory fluid losses. This is further compounded by the fact that aerobic performance is impaired to a greater extent at a high altitude for the same amount of dehydration (fluid lost), which necessitates assessment of both hydration status and increased fluid needs (Sawka, Cheuvront, and Kenefick 2015). On the flip side, athletes training or racing in a hot, dry climate will have decreased sweat rates and therefore may not require as much total fluid to meet their hydration needs. See table 9.5 for a summary of athletes' fluid needs during exercise.

Incidence of rhabdomyolysis (rapid breakdown of damaged skeletal muscle tissue) is also increased with dehydration and can lead to pain, vomiting, confusion, irregular heartbeat, and eventually kidney failure if the athlete is not treated and rehydrated. Due to all of the above facts about hydration

TABLE 9.5   Fluid Intake Guidelines During Exercise

Goals	Guideline (how to)	Starting point	Notes
Replace fluid lost to sweat during exercise to minimize dehydration to <2% body weight Do not exceed sweat loss to minimize risk of hyponatremia	Customize your fluid replacement plan based on sweat rate testing	0.4-0.8 L/hr (14-27 oz/hr) Increase (or decrease) as needed based on your individual sweat rate, climate, and acclimatization	Sweat rates vary widely between athletes, for individual athletes throughout the season, and depending on acclimatization Include sodium (sport drink or other source) if you are a salty sweater, sweat >1.2L/hr (>40 oz/hr), are training or competing for more than two hours, or exercising in a hot environment

Spotlight on Meghan Newcomer

Meghan Newcomer excelled in swimming and soccer early on, then quickly became an internationally ranked triathlete. Her impressive athletic history includes a podium finish at Collegiate Triathlon Nationals representing Columbia University, a silver medal at Age Group Triathlon World Championships in Budapest, Hungry, representing the United States, and the Ironman World Championship in Hawaii. Meghan has also completed the World Marathon Challenge (i.e., seven marathons on seven continents in seven days) and countless other world athletic adventures. She's done all this while balancing her career as a physician's assistant in a busy New York City operating room.

How did you figure out and adapt to your high sweat rate?

In my early triathlon years, I would win a race and end up in the emergency room, or black out 2 miles before the finish line because of hydration issues. The first time it happened I thought it was a fluke and figured I just didn't hydrate well enough, but then it happened again, and it was pretty scary. It got to the point that I thought I was not going to be able to race again in the heat. That is when I came to see you. I finally went to a lab to do sweat rate testing in a heat chamber. We had suspected it but found out definitively that I am both a heavy sweater and salty sweater, and that my core temperature rises very quickly. They had to legally stop my test when my core temperature reached 107. I had been going from training in New York City to racing in Hawaii or Florida, and since it takes 21 days for your body to acclimate, I was literally running into trouble. On a hot day I lose over 5 pounds of fluid on a 45-minute run, which is impossible to get in (or absorb). We developed a plan where I did salt loading and also exposed my body to heat (in a sauna or steam room) for 21 days prior to hot-weather events. I'd sit there reading a book and hydrating with Himalayan sea salt in lemon water. I did this heat acclimatization training before each big race in the heat, and each time, my heart rate would jump up quickly and I would initially feel like I needed to get of the sauna or steam room ASAP. I started with 15 uncomfortable minutes and eventually was able to sit longer and longer more comfortably. A couple key points on this for anyone who wants to try it are that I started with a short amount of time and worked up to longer sessions, and I always focus on starting well hydrated and drinking while I am in the sauna or steam room.

How do you balance demanding work in the operating room with your training and nutrition?

It has been quite a challenge over the past three years, but I finally have it figured out. We may operate until ten o'clock on a Friday night, and since we can't eat or drink in the OR, I then miss the time I would normally eat dinner. At first this left me almost feeling hungover for my long workout on Saturday. I had to adjust to the craziness of my schedule and started bringing easy-to-eat carbs, including squeezable fruit and protein pouches, because I can suck them down quickly between cases. I also make Japanese rice balls with extra salt and nutrient-dense smoothies (with almond milk, banana, peanut butter, and protein), plus I eat an energy bar. It takes a bit of planning, but I can feel that it makes a big difference in my training and races, so I make it happen.

How else has your nutrition changed over your years as an elite athlete?

When I was younger, if for some reason I didn't get to eat as much as I should have before a morning workout I would still feel fine, but that is no longer the case. I was also definitely not as good about my recovery nutrition earlier in my athletic career, but now I plan in advance to make sure I have what I need—plenty of carbohydrate plus some protein. Again, working in the OR, it is even more important, since I never really know when I will be able to eat again. I also realized I needed to figure out what works for me—to test more things out for myself. I saw early on that each pro triathlete may have her way of eating, but there is no one right way to eat and no one food choice that will make or break your race or health. That was an important realization.

Have you changed your long-training and race-day fueling?

As I have gotten a bit older, I have become more comfortable paying attention to what I crave. For example, I once drank an entire bottle of pickle juice in the longest single-day bike race in the United States, called Logan to Jackson. Because of my high fluid and high salt needs, I want (and need) salty foods, and I honor that. I make ginger sushi rice balls, which always appeal to me.

What is your intake like for ultraendurance events?

In 2018 I did the world marathon challenge, which, as it turns out, I was unknowingly "training" for with my erratic work schedule, in terms of eating, running, and sleeping at all different times. Traveling around the world running marathons came with its own set of nutritional challenges. We didn't have time to buy food, didn't always have the foods we wanted, and were constantly trying to eat to recover and also to digest enough food to get us ready for the next marathon. I ended up eating a lot of potato chips, because they had salt and seemed to digest easily, and of course we couldn't bring bananas and other fruits, because they would be confiscated going through customs in different countries.

How big of a role do you think nutrition plays in athletic performance for Masters athletes?

There is no such thing as the best diet or a cheat day or the ability to think, "Uh-oh, my race is coming up, so I should eat well now." When I was younger, I would only focus on my nutrition the day before the race and the day of the race. Now I try to establish overall good principles and then, as I approach a big event, recognize that I need to eat more carbs to fuel my heavier training load and make those adjustments.

Meghan's Favorite Postrace Meal

I don't have anything I always eat after a race. Since I do so much international racing, I just like to be adventurous after races. I like to try whatever the country I'm in is known for.

and the importance of sodium balance in our bodies, the IOM recommends consuming "sports beverages" containing 20 to 30 milliequivalents per liter of sodium during hot weather and longer-duration (>2 hr) exercise.

Athletes with high total sweat losses and fluid intake needs should develop a plan to ensure they are meeting both their fluid and sodium needs but not exceeding their carbohydrate absorption capabilities. This plan should include consumption of a mixture of sport drinks containing carbohydrate as well as water throughout training sessions and competitions (Maughan and Shirreffs 2008). Diluting sport drinks is not generally recommended, because that will decrease both carbohydrate and sodium intake as well as decrease fluid absorption rate.

What Athletes Need to Know About Hyponatremia

Excessive fluid intake (drinking more than the total of sweat and urine losses) can lead to hyponatremia, a condition marked by the dilution of blood sodium concentration to less than 135 millimoles per liter. This is generally a result of excessive total sodium loss and excessive consumption of water or low-sodium fluid prior to or during the event. While not as common as dehydration in athletes, the risk of hyponatremia can be acutely dangerous. Symptoms include headache, bloating, puffiness (especially in the hands and feet), weight gain during exercise, nausea, vomiting, headaches, con-fusion, disorientation, seizures, respiratory distress, loss of consciousness, and death if not recognized and treated with medical attention right away. Athletes at higher risk for hyponatremia include smaller individuals and those with lower sweat rates who are exercising for long durations of time (>4 hours) (ACSM et al. 2007). It is important to note that it is possible for an athlete to be both dehydrated and hyponatremic, as is sometimes seen in marathoners, endurance athletes, and football players.

Why Muscle Cramping Occurs and What a Masters Athlete Can Do About It

The true causes of muscle cramping have been debated over recent years. While it is now accepted that some muscle cramps are the result of muscle fatigue, many others are attributed to dehydration and electrolyte imbalances, especially in salty sweaters and athletes with high sweat rates (Thomas, Erdman, and Burke 2016). Athletes in all sports—but specifically tennis, American football, and endurance athletes, who are prone to muscle cramp-ing—can reduce the frequency and duration of muscle cramps by ingesting both water and salt (Maughan and Shirreffs 2008). Athletes should monitor their fluid loss during exercise and assess sodium loss in sweat as able, then attempt to increase sodium intake to match their losses. For athletes with particularly high sodium sweat content, beverages with higher sodium concentration than a normal sport drink way be warranted (Maughan and Shirreffs 2008). For many performance athletes, sweat rates frequently exceed fluid intake and should be matched as closely as possible (within fluid access constraints and fluid absorption rates) to minimize fluid loss to less than 2 percent of body weight during exercise, then fully replenished upon completion of the exercise session or competition. For athletes in sports where ad lib drinking is not allowed (e.g., tennis, American football, soccer), athletes need to encourage themselves and their teammates to take advantage of drinking opportunities when they arise (e.g., between sets, during time-outs, at halftime) to prevent dehydration and muscle cramping.

Postexercise Rehydration

In general, fluid balance can be returned to normal with adequate food and fluid intake during the 8 to 24 hours following an exercise session (ACSM et al. 2007). In order to restore euhydration during this time, athletes need to drink 125 to 150 percent of total fluid lost to sweat during exercise over the six hours immediately following completion of exercise (Shirreffs 1996). (See table 9.6 for postexercise fluid guidelines.) In addition, following strenuous or prolonged exercise sessions, plain water will not be as effective at rehydrating as a food or beverage containing sodium and may not correct the fluid deficit as efficiently. Studies show that attempting to rehydrate with plain water alone (and without salty foods to help the body hold on to much-needed water) only serves to decrease the drive to drink, and stimulates urine output, which can prolong the period of time to restore fluid balance by three times (Shirreffs et al. 1996). The ACSM Position Statement (ACSM et al. 2007) says that fully replacing fluid and electrolyte deficits may require "aggressive" rehydration depending on the magnitude of the deficit and goal and timing of the next session. After exercise, athletes can often tolerate beverages with high sodium concentrations and should be allowed and encouraged to self-select such beverages as long as they are palatable to promote optimal rehydration for each individual (Shirreffs 1996). If an athlete has less than 12 hours to recover between sessions, he will need to actively

TABLE 9.6 Postexercise Fluid Intake Guidelines

Goal	Guidelines (how to)	Time frame	Notes
Replace fluid lost to sweat during exercise	Athletes must replace 125-150% of fluid lost during each session within 2 hours postexercise Drink 1.25-1.50 L of fluid per kg of body weight (20-24 oz/lb) lost during exercise	Within four to six hours after training session or competition	Include fluids and foods with salt to taste to help stimulate thirst and promote rehydration and fluid retention

Spotlight on Gail Waesche Kislevitz

Gail Waesche Kislevitz is a 27-time marathoner, running coach, and acclaimed author of many sports and fitness books, including *The Spirit of the Marathon, First Marathons, First Triathlons* and her latest book, *Running Past Fifty*. In 2018, she finished the Tokyo Marathon and was awarded the World Marathon Majors Medal, signifying she had completed all six world major marathons. Gail has been a runner for more than 50 years and has coached for the New York Road Runners (NYRR) charity program, Team for Kids. Gail spoke to me about her hydration and fueling, and opened up about her past struggle with anorexia nervosa, describing how her love of running allowed her to begin fueling again and move on.

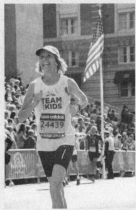

© Gail Waesche Kislevitz

How has your nutrition and hydration intake changed over your years as a Masters runner?

When I started running more than 50 years ago, there were no guidelines at all and no sports products available. No one was talking about nutrition or hydration for endurance athletes. Then slowly, guidelines came out about what runners should do, but it wasn't until I started racing in my 40s that I really started to pay attention and follow the guidelines. Now, as I get older, I find that I need to fuel more, and I definitely can't run on an empty stomach anymore.

How have your hydration needs changed as a Masters athlete?

Hydration is one area I have paid a lot more attention to as I have gotten older. When I was younger, I remember running marathons in 80-degree weather, thinking, "That's not so bad." Now at age 67, running in the heat is a lot more difficult, so I drink a lot more water when I'm out there, and I pay close attention to it. When you came to speak to our marathoners for the NYRR Team for Kids teams, you stressed the importance of hydration. From that, plus personal experience, I know that during a marathon or long run I have to drink before I am thirsty, and I always make sure to start getting fluid in early. Even though I don't sweat a lot, I run marathons, so it adds up, and I am very serious about my hydration.

Can you tell us about how and why you say that running saved your life?

I feel it is important to speak about fueling, and I am very willing to talk about my past eating disorder. I've talked about it in my own book. I had been running for years and was in therapy for anorexia for two to three years, and the therapist kept trying to find the key that would help us unravel it, that would be the "aha" moment. Eventually, and ironically, my decision to train for a marathon became that key. It gave me something more powerful than the disease itself. Of course, everyone thought I was absolutely out of my mind, and I understood their concern; I didn't eat. They literally thought I was going to die out there. But as a runner, I knew that in order to complete a marathon, I had to fuel, I had to eat. I had to do all those things that I had pretty much stopped doing when I developed anorexia. As a runner who was and is very passionate about what I do, that passion is what helped me get over the anorexia, which is so all-powerful and encompassing that it takes over your whole life. I started fueling in small doses. I remember the first time I sat down to eat a sandwich. I thought, "Well, I'll start here," and I couldn't. I ate maybe half the sandwich, and then I realized it was going to be a bigger challenge than I had thought. But I started eating in small increments. Every day I was eating a little bit more, and a little bit more, until I felt that I was not going to compromise myself through picking up distance running. I had maintained my running throughout my battle with anorexia, but now that I wanted that bigger challenge, I upped my carbs, and I upped my protein. As I added running mileage, I would make sure I was coming back and feeling healthy, not weak or light-headed; I "fueled" to be able to do my run and function thereafter. After I ran that marathon, I really did feel better about myself, and healthier eating continued sort of naturally. For me, running has been the key that made me eat better, and being part of the running community has been so important. After a race, I'd go out to brunch with a group of like-minded runner friends. On my own, I might just eat a muffin, but when I see other runners digging into stacks of pancakes and three eggs and having so much fun, then I am able to say that I too am going to order those pancakes because there's nothing wrong with it. There is a healthiness in being around other runners who have more of a normal appetite, a normal way of eating and looking at food. That's a good lesson.

How do you feel about statements and perceptions that thinner equals faster?

It is terribly unfortunate when an athlete is really enjoying a sport and wants to get better, to then hear someone say that getting thinner will get her there. Coaches and teammates need to be aware of this and stop perpetuating this, because if an athlete gets caught up in losing too much weight, then it can be hard to get out. There are many consequences of underfueling.

Can eating more equal thinner and faster?

Many pro runners are now on social media or writing cookbooks, talking about how they love to eat. They are fueling well and adequately because they are smart, because they haven't gotten caught up in it all. It is motivating because I know they must be doing it right.

Do you have any words of wisdom for others struggling with fueling their bodies or with an eating disorder?

Absolutely. Here is what works for me:

- Running is important to my life.
- Running is my passion.
- I have to fuel my body.
- I have to take care of my body.

Gail's Favorite Postrace Meal

It's not a meal, but what I usually really want is a good chocolate chip cookie.

seek to rehydrate by taking in 1.5 liters of fluid per kilogram of body weight (23 oz/lb) lost to sweat during exercise over the first six hours immediately after completion of exercise. Failure to replace sodium as well as fluids only leads to increased urine production rather than rehydration.

So, the next time your recovery time is short and you have another important session coming up soon (<12 hours), be sure to take in some salty drinks and foods in order to stimulate your thirst, help your body hold on to the fluids you drink (and eat), and return your plasma volume to normal in order to fully rehydrate before you start sweating again. Excessive alcohol should be avoided during this recovery period because it acts as a diuretic and will only worsen your rehydration problem. Caffeine, on the other hand, and contrary to popular belief, when consumed at less than 180 milligrams, can generally be considered part of your total rehydration (Thomas, Erdman, and Burke 2016).

The bottom line is that there is wide variation in sweat rate, sodium content of sweat, and therefore fluid and salt needs both between and among individual athletes. Generalized fluid recommendations will not meet the need of many athletes. Sweat and salt measurements should be taken as previously described, and athletes should take responsibility to understand and meet their unique and ever-changing fluid and hydration needs in order to optimize performance and overall health outcomes. As athletes, we should get in the habit of paying attention to our thirst, urine color and amount, and weight loss due to sweat during exercise, and make adjustments in fluid and sodium intake according to changes that we see before, during, or after training and during our usual daily life. Any athlete who notices weight gain during training or competition should assess whether it is accompanied by a large volume of pale or clear urine (a sign of over-drinking during exercise) or whether they might have been dehydrated before they started (confirmed by low volume of or darker-than-usual urine before exercise) and simply made up that loss (Maughan and Shirreffs 2008). Athletes who have ascertained that they are salty sweaters should consider beverages with higher sodium content or adding salt to foods before, during (as appropriate), and after exercise, and note whether their high sodium loss is contributing to muscle cramping (Maughan and Shirreffs 2008).

On the previous pages, you heard athlete and author Gail Waesche Kislevitz talk about everything from her changing fluid needs as a Masters athlete to how training for a marathon helped her learn to fuel her body and overcome anorexia. Gail's story is a perfect segue into chapter 10, in which we will discuss what I call the slippery slope of underfueling. Whether you or anyone you know has ever struggled with underfueling, an eating disorder, body image issues, or a less-than-ideal relationship with food, this next chapter will help you see the importance of understanding our complex relationships with food, weight, and body image.

10 | Underfueling

Do you remember when and why you first started participating in athletics? You might have been a school-age child with boundless energy whose parents encouraged you to get out and play. You might not have picked up sports until later in life for reasons that range from improving your health, increasing energy, boosting mood, losing weight, or a whole host of other benefits. This chapter is about another side of sport that, as a sports dietitian for more than 15 years, I have seen all too often: underfueling and disordered eating in athletes.

If you have been in athletics for a while, you may already be familiar with the term *female athlete triad*, which was first identified in 1992. Before we examine the female athlete triad and what is now referred to as relative energy deficiency in sport (RED-S), it is important to take the time to explain the prevalence, signs, and symptoms of eating disorders, both in the general population and in athletes.

Defining Eating Disorders

Eating disorders (ED) are often misunderstood, underreported, and underdiagnosed. They are serious but treatable illnesses that fall under the heading of mental illness and manifest in both physical and physiological ways; all body systems are adversely affected by consistent undereating and underfueling. ED affect both females and males across all races, ethnicities, socioeconomic statuses, and ages, and are seen at a disproportionality high rate among athletes. ED are associated with severe disturbances in

---

Before we delve into the important topic of underfueling in athletes, I want to start by saying that if the information in this chapter causes you to question your food behaviors or those of someone you know, please check out the National Eating Disorders Association (NEDA) website at www.nationaleatingdisorders.org for lists of signs, symptoms, and diagnosis criteria for specific eating disorders; an easy-to-use screening tool; as well as resources for professionals including therapists, dietitians, and physicians who are trained and ready to help.

both food intake and emotions and thoughts about food, body image, and body size. Once thought to be found mostly in adolescents, eating disorders have been increasingly seen in older adults. A national survey estimates that 20 million women and 1 million men in the United States will have an ED at some point in their lives. And while there is no one known cause for ED, a growing consensus suggests that a range of biological, psychological, and sociocultural factors contribute to their development. The combination of emotional and physical components found in ED must be treated to avoid their many serious complications, which are widespread throughout the body and can include malnutrition, heart problems and electrolyte imbalances, and other serious and sometimes fatal conditions. Treatment for athletes with these mental illnesses ideally involves a team consisting of at least a medical doctor, psychologist, and sports dietitian.

Throughout this chapter I will discuss the progression, dangers, and treatment of ED. I will also introduce you to two athletes to help me shed light on this tricky-to-explain and often difficult-to-comprehend topic: Ellen Hart, who will walk you through what it feels like to live with and compete at a high level while battling an ED, and Stephanie Roth Goldberg, an endurance athlete and sports psychotherapist who works with athletes with ED to help them redefine their relationship with food and their bodies.

Ellen's story is so poignant and relevant that I share much of the rest of it throughout the chapter; it's too important for only a single sidebar.

There is a higher incidence of ED among athletes versus non athletes of all ages, and this includes Masters athletes. Since ED are often difficult to identify and diagnose, there is a wide range of stated incidence of occurrence. But there is known to be a significant link between exercise compulsion and ED behavior. For example, 40 to 80 percent of those diagnosed with anorexia nervosa (AN) are said to use excessive exercise as a way to help them avoid weight gain (NEDA 2018), and a shocking 3 out of 10 people seeking weight loss exhibit signs of binge eating disorder (BED). Weight-class athletes such as those in wrestling, rowing, and horse racing and those in aesthetic sports such as gymnastics, swimming, and bodybuilding have even higher rates of ED, often quoted as high as 63 percent. It is largely assumed that ED only affect women, but 25 percent of people diagnosed with AN and 40 percent of those diagnosed with BED are males.

We'll now discuss the signs, symptoms, and risks for AN, BN, BED, and orthorexia. I include references if you wish to learn more.

Anorexia Nervosa

AN is an eating disorder characterized by restricted energy intake relative to energy requirements, a fear of weight gain, and body image distortion or denial of the seriousness of underfueling or being underweight. Many with AN will restrict food groups and food types, and consider many foods off limits. It is important to note that you cannot always tell when a person is struggling with AN. Athletes with AN may be consuming what initially appears to be a substantial amount of food but remains much less than their total daily energy needs. AN is not really about food. It develops as an unhealthy attempt to cope with emotional issues in which thinness comes to equal self-worth. It can be a life-threatening conditioning that requires early detection and much support.

Atypical AN includes those individuals who meet the criteria for AN but who are not underweight despite significant weight loss.

Individuals with AN may exhibit any or all of the following symptoms:

- Preoccupation with food, weight, calories, and dieting
- Avoidance of mealtimes and situations involving food
- Limited or decreased social interactions
- Strong need for control
- Inflexible thinking about food and refusal to eat whole food groups or categories
- Excessive and rigid exercise regimes despite obstacles including weather, illness, and injury
- Denial of feeling hungry
- Disturbance in the way one experiences or perceives his or her body shape and weight
- Dramatic weight loss
- Intense fear of gaining weight

Over time, the following symptoms may develop as the body goes into starvation:

- Menstrual irregularities including amenorrhea
- Osteopenia or osteoporosis (thinning of the bones) through loss of calcium
- Brittle hair and nails
- Stomach cramping, severe constipation, acid reflux, etc.
- Poor wound healing and impaired immune function
- Drop in blood pressure, heart rate, thyroid function, and hormone levels
- Mood disturbance including depression and anxiety
- Fine hair on body (lanugo)

To further highlight the complexity of this disease, two-thirds of those with AN have been found to exhibit signs of anxiety disorder years prior to their ED diagnosis and often exhibit qualities including perfectionism, obsessive-compulsive traits, and concern about following rules or fear of making mistakes (NEDA 2018).

Spotlight on Ellen Hart

Ellen Hart (Peña) is an elite endurance athlete who qualified for the 1980 Olympic trials in the 10,000 meter and competed in the Olympic marathon trials in 1984 before coming to terms with and eventually going public with her battle with bulimia nervosa. She once held the U.S. record for the 30-kilometer and the world record for the 20-kilometer. She earned a BA from Harvard and a law degree from the University of Colorado Law School. In the past 12 years, she has returned to competitive endurance sports with gusto as a triathlete and has, as she said, "managed to snag" 18 age-group world championships in all triathlon distances. Among those, Ellen has won her age group in the Ironman World Championship in Kona, Hawaii, three times and the Ironman 70.3 World Championship seven times. She is passionate about spreading the word about and helping others struggling with ED, and I am forever grateful to her for openly and honestly sharing her story with us all.

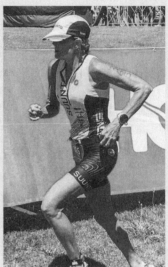

Photo by Cary Craig 2019.

When and how did your eating disorder start?

When I was growing up, food was just food. You liked and ate certain things and not others, and that was that. Then in ninth grade I started to think seriously about running, and I started to restrict my eating. I really did think that one calorie was the same as the next calorie, and that if I had a caloric deficit, that was a good day. That's when my periods stopped, because I was under my weight set-point that my body needed to be fertile. My mom was concerned and took me to the doctor, who gave me a shot that got my period going again. Then I stopped running and played team sports with my sister, and I was fine for the rest of high school and almost all of college.

When did you get bitten by the running bug?

During my freshman year in college in Boston, I went to see the Boston Marathon with my roommate, and I still remember watching and feeling the hair on my arms stand up because it was so exciting to me that people were running this marathon event. And somewhere in the back of my mind I thought, "I want to do this!"

I was running for Harvard, and during my junior year of college I also started really training for the marathon. I had to run a full marathon under the qualifying time in order to be able to run the Boston marathon. I ran a marathon in March in 3:11, then ran Boston in 3:06 and really liked it. My track coach had threatened to kick me off the track team if I ran the marathon, but I really wanted to run it, so I did, and they didn't let me compete on the track team that spring.

How do you feel when you hear people say that lighter equals faster?

To be honest, that whole time I always felt like I was a few pounds overweight, but I never did anything about it until my senior year of college. I was running indoor winter track when my coach said, "You should lose a little bit of weight and you'll run faster," and I did, at first in mostly healthy ways. Then a bit later he said, "It looks like you have gained some of the weight back," and right then and there, there was some click in my brain, some horrible click that really solidified things that had been going on for years, and I thought, "I will never ever let him or anyone else ever say that or think that about me ever again." Then I started down the horrible road of an eating disorder.

What was it like to run competitively while battling an ED?

I would restrict my eating, but then of course couldn't do it forever, so I would eat something that I thought I wasn't supposed to, and that would turn into a binge, because if I had eaten one bad thing, I might as well eat 20 more things. And I kept thinking that I was in control, but after about a year I realized I was not in control and that I could not stop. From there it got progressively worse. Overall, that pattern lasted 10 years. Back then there was no one to find on the internet, no way to search for treatments or specialists who worked with people with ED. I had nowhere to turn for help.

During the first five years it was pretty much just self-loathing isolation. I went to law school but interrupted that schooling in order to train for the 1984 Olympic marathon, which had just been added to the Olympic schedule. I started individual and group treatment, therapy, meditation, basically anything I thought might help, but nothing helped. I had some good finish times: I ran a 2:35 marathon and a 32:42 10k, but I never reached my full potential at either distance because I was injured all the time from not fueling myself properly.

How did your eating disorder affect your relationships and public image?

I was married to the mayor of Denver and, on the outside, I was going to parties and looking healthy and happy, and everyone knew me as "Ellen the runner." But I was a fraud.

In public, I was the happy, healthy runner, and I would tell interviewers, "You don't want to interview me; trust me, you don't want me." And as they were interviewing me, I was thinking, "Do you really want to know what I do? No, you don't."

The fraud piece was really damaging to me emotionally, spiritually, and in terms of self-confidence coming up to the 1984 marathon trials. I had American and world records and a legitimate shot at making the Olympic team, and I knew that. So I thought six months prior to the trials that if I could just not be bulimic for six months, I could really make this team. Then six months slipped to three months, then one month, then one week, and I never could stop. Going into the marathon trials I was obviously not as prepared nutritionally and physically as I should have been. And, of course, that was pretty damaging psychologically.

Out of about 260 women who qualified to run the trials I finished eleventh, which I can look back on now and say was good, but it was eight places out from where I wanted to be to make the Olympic team.

I ran for another year then completely fell apart. My body was depleted and wasted. It was really hellish. By then I had graduated from law school and had a really good job with a really good firm, but all I could think about was eating. Not really eating, but bingeing and purging. I didn't know what it was like to be hungry and I didn't know what it felt like to be full, but from when my eyelids popped open in the morning until my head hit the pillow at night that was all I was thinking about. Every day I would think, "OK, maybe today I can be disciplined and maybe I can control this," and I couldn't.

Anorexia Athletica

A condition related to AN, anorexia athletica is a sports-specific subclinical ED that was first identified in 1983 (Bär and Markser 2013). Its definition has since been widened to include many indices including weight loss, caloric restriction, and fear of gaining weight. It has been shown that more than 73 percent of athletes across various sports demonstrated at least one criteria of an eating disorder (Bär and Markser 2013), and as such all individuals working with athletes need to be knowledgeable about the warning signs, performance effects, referral sources, and necessary treatment.

Bulimia Nervosa

BN is characterized by a repeated cycle of bingeing and subsequent compensatory behavior such as purging or excessive exercise. A general lack of control over food intake or type is often described during binge eating, while compensatory behaviors can range from self-induced vomiting to laxative use to excessive exercise in an attempt to prevent weight gain or as punishment. Diagnosis requires at least one episode of bingeing and purging per week for at least three months.

It is important to note that the foundation for ED is often laid early in life; 40 to 60 percent of girls ages 6 to 12 are already concerned with becoming fat. A history of dieting has been found to increase one's risk of developing an ED five-fold, while "extreme dieting" has been associated with an 18-fold increased risk of developing an ED (NEDA 2018). Another important note is that a high rate of individuals with BN also struggle with substance abuse, self-injury (cutting), and impulsivity as other forms of self-punishment.

Individuals with BN may exhibit any or all of the following symptoms:

- Binges in which the amount of food eaten is larger than most people would eat in a similar amount of time and under similar circumstances
- Feeling a lack of control over the amount or type of food eaten
- Development of food rituals such as eating only particular foods and adhering to food rules and restrictions
- Concern with behaviors indicting attempts at weight loss, dieting, and control of food intake
- Lack of comfort or willingness to eat with others or taking very small portions of food when eating with others
- Skipping meals and irregular meal patterns
- Extreme mood swings
- Evidence of binge eating including empty wrappers or containers, disappearance of large amounts of food, or hoarding food
- Evidence of inappropriate compensatory behavior including frequent trips to the bathroom after meals or other signs or smells

Over time, the following symptoms may develop:

- Anemia and depressed thyroid and hormone levels
- Low potassium
- Slowed heart rate
- Weight within normal or overweight range
- Difficulty concentrating
- Calluses across tops of fingers as a result of vomiting
- Brittle nails and thinning hair
- Muscle weakness and cold or swollen feet
- Menstrual irregularities including amenorrhea
- Poor wound healing and depressed immune function

On the previous pages, you heard Ellen Hart discuss how her ED developed into BN and how she continued to run while battling her ED until she no longer could. While Ellen struggled with BN for a decade of her early life, others develop a pattern of uncontrolled eating and feeling out of control with food and eating without the compensatory behaviors. They express a severe lack of control over the amount or type of food eaten during a binge episode, and often cannot or do not stop eating until they are way beyond uncomfortably full. This pattern is called binge eating disorder (BED).

Binge Eating Disorder

BED is characterized by the consumption of larger than normal quantities of food over a short period of time (generally two hours). It is associated with a loss of control over one's eating, eating rapidly even when not hungry, and not being able to stop eating despite discomfort. It is diagnosed when the bingeing occurs an average of at least once per week for at least three months. It is different from BN in that regular compensatory behaviors are not present. BED is the most common eating disorder in the United States and is often accompanied by feelings of shame, guilt, and depression.

Individuals with BED may exhibit any or all of the following symptoms:

- Statement of or appearance of being uncomfortable around food and eating
- Feelings of disgust, depression, guilt, or distress after overeating
- Low self-esteem
- Large weight fluctuations
- Lack of control when eating during binge episodes
- Stealing or hoarding large quantities of food
- Erratic eating behaviors including skipped meals, repetitive fasting, and cyclic dieting

Over time, the following symptoms may develop:

- Rapid weight fluctuations, both up and down
- Stomach upset such as cramping, constipation, and reflux
- Difficulty concentrating

Orthorexia

Although orthorexia is not officially recognized as a diagnosable ED, it deserves our attention. The term *orthorexia* was coined in 1998 and is characterized by an obsession with eating what one perceives as healthfully to the point of it being a detriment to one's health. The most recent term for this is *eating clean*. As a sports dietitian, I see this condition in athletes all too often, and many try to claim, or truly believe that this über-healthy eating is part of "being serious about my sport." Without official criteria to diagnose, and per the athlete's report of eating to performance, this disordered eating pattern often goes unrecognized for a long time in athletes until it has become severe enough to affect performance and recovery or the overall health of the athlete. Although many people think it initially sounds harmless or even virtuous, orthorexia generally results in an unhealthy relationship with food, guilt about eating anything one does not perceive as "perfectly healthy," and underfueling due to refusal to eat a wide range of foods. Individuals with orthorexia often also exhibit symptoms of anxiety around food, social isolation, and ignoring hunger cues and intuition about eating. Orthorexia can lead to malnutrition due to refusal to eat many foods the individual has inaccurately labeled "unhealthy."

Individuals with orthorexia may exhibit any or all of the following symptoms:

- Refusal to eat all but a narrow group of "healthy" foods
- Excessive thinking, speaking, writing, and reading about healthy foods and lifestyle
- Excessive thinking about what is safe or healthy to eat
- Compulsively checking ingredient lists and nutrition labels

Over time, an individual with orthorexia who is underfueling and energy deficient will also show symptoms similar to those seen in AN due to restriction of food variety, type, and overall intake. In our current world of social media, where anyone can post their opinions about food, exercise, and what is healthy, whether they are qualified or not, this unhealthy eating pattern is often difficult to uncover.

Energy Availability in Athletes

The female athlete triad (see figure 10.1) was originally characterized by the presence of three things—disordered eating, amenorrhea (absence of

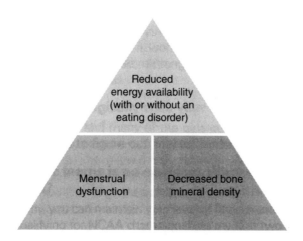

FIGURE 10.1 The female athlete triad.

menstruation), and osteoporosis (Otis et al. 1997). Since the term was first coined, the female athlete triad has come to be known as a more elaborate range of interconnected conditions related to underfueling and disordered eating. In 2007 the American College of Sports Medicine (ACSM) published a position stand by Nattiv et al. that referred to the triad as an "interrelationship among energy availability, menstrual function and bone mineral density, which may have clinical manifestations including eating disorders, functional hypothalamic amenorrhea, and osteoporosis" (page 1867).

As implied by the name, the female athlete triad did not recognize the importance of the prevalence of low energy availability in male athletes. Because of this and other considerations, the International Olympic Committee (IOC) introduced a new name with broader reach in 2014: relative energy deficiency in sport (RED-S), the definition of which was updated again in 2018 to include a better understanding of measuring and quantifying of low energy availability, greater acknowledgement and understanding of RED-S in male athletes, and performance parameters affected by RED-S (Mountjoy et al. 2018). RED-S refers to "impaired physiological functioning caused by relative energy deficiency and includes, but is not limited to, impairments of metabolic rate, menstrual function, bone health, immunity, protein synthesis and cardiovascular health" (page 687). (See figure 10.2.)

In ACSM's definition, energy availability is defined as nutritional intake minus exercise expenditure, and low energy availability (defined as less than 30 kcal/kg [14 kcal/lb] of fat-free mass [FFM] per day) is said to be the factor that leads to impairments in both reproductive and skeletal health. The original female athlete triad was broadened so that an athlete may be diagnosed if any of the three are present. The position statement explains that due to the high incidence and severe nature of the consequences of prolonged decreased energy availability, all athletes should be screened for

Relative energy deficiency in sport (RED-S)

Effects on health	
Gastrointestinal issues	Development and growth
Immune function	Hematological effects
Cardiovascular function	Metabolic disruption
Menstrual irregularities ⎫ Part of female	Endocrine function
Bone health ⎭ athlete triad	Psychological impact*

Effects on performance	
Less endurance	Depression
Higher risk of injury	Impaired judgment
Lower muscle strength	Irritability
Decreased storage of glycogen	Reduced coordination
Hampered training response	Reduced concentration

FIGURE 10.2 Relative energy deficiency in sport (RED-S) can affect both health and sport performance. *Psychological consequences can either precede or result from RED-S.

Adapted from Mountjoy et al. (2018).

the triad at a preparticipation physical or annual health exam or whenever any athlete presents with any of the signs or symptoms associated with it. Payne and Kitchener (2014) recommend including orthostatic blood pressure measurement and BMI calculation and looking for physical signs of ED including cold extremities, lanugo, knuckle scars, or parotid gland enlargement in the physical screening of athletes. Once the triad is suspected or identified, a multidisciplinary team is recommended, including a physician, a registered dietitian well versed in working with athletes with ED, and a mental health practitioner, and should have the common primary goal of increasing energy intake and reducing exercise energy expenditure.

For Masters athletes, no pre-participation physical is generally required to sign up for a marathon, join a swim team, or play with a local soccer club. Therefore, it becomes even more important for everyone in the athletic community to be aware of the signs and symptoms of disordered eating and low energy availability in athletes and to know what to do if they suspect a friend, teammate, athlete, or loved one needs help. Of course, it makes sense that athletes with an ED have an eight-times higher risk of injury versus athletes who do not have an ED, and it is during those times of diagnosis and treatment of an athlete's injury that opportunity to screen and then treat for eating disorders and disordered eating often arises.

Although this chapter is mostly about ED in athletes, it is important to acknowledge that sometimes low energy availability is simply the result of an athlete's unintentional failure to increase nutritional intake to meet the high energy demands of training. Unlike with true ED, whose road to optimal intake and recovery is often long and winding, when an energy mismatch develops as training load increases and does not involve an ED, the athlete is generally quick to correct the problem and increase their intake once it is discovered. Ben Kessel's story on the next page is an example of just that.

Consequences of Low Energy Availability

The effects of low energy availability are far reaching and include many hormonal changes that are likely the body's way of attempting to conserve energy when not enough is available for important bodily functions essential for life. These include but are not limited to altered thyroid function; decreased leptin and increased ghrelin (key appetite-regulating hormones); decreased insulin, growth hormone, and testosterone; and increased cortisol (a stress hormone). Many para-athletes are already at higher than average risk for impaired bone health due to decreased skeletal loading, may have alterations in baseline menstrual function if central neurological injury has occurred, may have either reduced energy needs due to decreased daily mobility or increased energy needs due to prosthetic use and gait asymmetry, and should also be screened for RED-S (Mountjoy et al. 2018).

The adverse health consequences of low energy availability on hormones and female menstrual function have been well studied and documented. Studies have shown that even a short-term, five-day energy deficit of less than 30 kilocalories per kilogram (14 kcal/lb) of FFM per day is enough to elicit decreases in hormone levels, and that the frequency and severity of menstrual disturbance is higher with increasing magnitude of the energy deficit (Mountjoy et al. 2018). The same study stated that extensive research in laboratory trials showed that in order to maintain healthy physiological function, optimal energy availability (EA) is typically achieved at 45 kilocalories per kilogram (20 kcal/lb) of FFM per day, and that many physiological systems are disrupted at EA less than 30 kilocalories per kilogram (14 kcal/lb) of FFM per day, which roughly equates to an individual's average RMR. That said, this numerical cutoff does not predict amenorrhea in all women and should be used as a guide and in conjunction with other signs and symptoms of RED-S. Furthermore, obtaining accurate records of intake and exercise expenditure from training and competition plus other recreational and lifestyle activity can be very challenging. Using specialized equipment to measure RMR and body composition are essential, as are motivation and honesty in the reporting of food intake by the athlete. These tools should also be used in combination with an in-person interview. The bottom line is that it is *never* OK for a female athlete to stop menstruation just because of her high training volume. If energy needs are met, mensuration can and will continue, which is a fact that must be stressed among athletes, coaches, and medical professionals.

The 2018 IOC consensus statement on RED-S explains numerous important additional considerations, including the following.

- Low energy availability has been correlated with low ferritin and iron deficiency anemia in female athletes.

- Low energy availability disrupts digestion and induces many gastrointestinal complaints in the underfueled athlete. Delayed gastric emptying, constipation, stool leakage, and increased intestinal transit time have all been reported. These are often wrongfully dismissed by athletes, coaches, and families, and not recognized as signs and symptoms of an underlying ED and low energy availability as they should be.

- Immunological function is also compromised for athletes in a low energy availability state. Higher rates of upper respiratory infections, lower antibody responses, and complaints of body ache and other symptoms have been shown in amenorrheic and underfueled athletes.

- Early onset of atherosclerosis has been associated with lower than normal estrogen levels in underfueled female athletes, while dyslipidemia and depressed heart rates are also seen in amenorrheic athletes. In more severe cases of AN, serious cardiac abnormalities can occur.

- Mood is often also adversely affected by low energy availability, and numerous studies have shown increased rates of depression, low self-esteem, anxiety and psychosomatic disorders, and a decreased ability to manage stress under such conditions. Higher drive for thinness scores on the Eating Disorder Inventory (EDI), which can be administered by a mental health professional, are also associated with lower resting energy expenditure (lower metabolic rate).

Spotlight on Ben Kessel

We return to the story of Ben Kessel (see chapter 6), because it is a perfect example of how an informed, accomplished, and well-intended athlete can fall prey to underfueling when training demands soar. Ben and I had already known and worked with each other professionally when he came to see me in 2014 while training for an Ironman Triathlon. He wanted to nail down his fluid, sodium, carb, and energy needs before his upcoming race in Cozumel, Mexico, where it was going to be hot. We decided to test his resting metabolic rate (RMR), which I expected would be above average due to his combined high training volume and high muscle mass, but to our surprise, the test showed that his RMR was about normal for his height and weight. After reviewing his food and training log, I figured out very quickly why this was the case—he had not managed to increase his overall nutritional intake in relation to his increased training load that season. Since Ben's low energy availability was not due to an ED, but to an unintentional but significant gap between his high total energy needs to support his Ironman training and nutritional intake,

Because many of the symptoms are difficult to see, the prevalence of ED among athletes is very difficult to assess, especially now that only one of three initial criteria need be present for diagnosis. In a review of 65 studies, Gibbs, Williams, and De Souza (2013) demonstrated this to be the case, showing that the prevalence of any one of the triad symptoms ranged from 16 percent to as high as 60 percent in exercising women and female athletes, while the prevalence of two of the conditions ranged from 2.7 to 27 percent, and the prevalence of all three ranged from 0 to 15.9 percent. Other work demonstrates that the rate of ED among elite female athletes is as high as 20 to 31 percent, compared with 5.5 to 9 percent of the general population (Mehta, Thompson, and Kling 2018). This study also states that secondary amenorrhea (the absence of menstrual bleeding in a woman who had previously been menstruating but later stopped for three or more months in the absence of pregnancy) is as high as 69 percent in studies of dancers and 65 percent in studies among female long-distance runners.

Low Energy Availability Prevalence in Male Athletes

Growing evidence shows that many male athletes experience low energy availability, or a mismatch between energy intake and training exercise expenditure, especially cyclists, rowers, runners, jockeys, and athletes in weight class sports. This can be caused by a multitude of factors including failure to increase voluntary intake to meet increased energy needs in high-expenditure sports such as endurance sports (e.g., marathoners, triathletes, ultramarathoners), inadequate food availability or food insecurity, or of course

he was physically and mentally able to adjust his intake quite quickly and raise his metabolic rate back to where it should have been within a few months.

How did you increase your resting metabolic rate?

When we tested my RMR, it was just average, and since I am 6'1", was 200 pounds, and training for an Ironman (IM), we were both surprised by this. It seemed that at the end of the day I just wasn't eating as many calories as I needed, and I wanted to make sure I was fueling my IM training, so I increased my intake as you asked me to. You recommended that I increase the total amount I was eating up to 3,400 calories per day. I did this from August until right after IM in December—and my metabolic rate went up 10 percent. Of course, I was thrilled about that, but even better than the immediate gratification was the long-lasting mental effect—thinking that I have this fire and I need to be fueling to keep the wood chips burning—was a really big deal for me. Seeing that direct cause and effect was a great lesson for me in my own training and gave me a lot of confidence to keep eating a lot, especially when I am training a lot.

disordered eating. Reductions in testosterone levels and RMR can be red flags for further investigation. Inability or unwillingness to increase food intake despite low RMR and body weight can indicate a need for further evaluation and referral.

Even though the definition of RED-S includes relative energy deficiency in both male and female athletes, ED, disordered eating, and exercise addiction are more likely to go unnoticed in males. Exercise dependence (EXD), also referred to as exercise addiction or compulsive exercise, involves uncontrolled excessive exercise, craving for physical training, and the inability of an individual to reduce his exercise amount despite risk of harmful consequences including injury, social isolation, and depression (Torstveit et al. 2019). This condition has been known to be associated with an ED and was studied by Torstveit and his colleagues to determine its relationship with RED-S in male endurance athletes. They looked at 53 trained long-distance runners, cyclists, and triathletes, ages 18 to 50 years, and found associations between higher exercise dependence scale scores and ED symptoms, biomarkers of RED-S, negative energy balance, and higher cortisol levels. They explained how male athletes in sports that emphasize leanness or measures such as the power-to-weight ratio in cycling are at increased risk for developing RED-S. They noted that reduced testosterone levels have been seen in male athletes following only five days of forced severe energy deficits. This energy deficiency can lead to long-term consequences affecting performance, increased muscle catabolism (breakdown) for use as an energy source, and overall negative health outcomes such as increased incidence of depression, higher cortisol and cholesterol levels, and reduced hormone levels. They recommended that once recognized, males with low energy availability be referred to a treatment team to assist them in increasing energy intake or reducing energy expenditure (exercise) to reverse the energy deficiency and risk of long-term complications.

In another study, 50 male competitive cyclists ages 18 to 71 were assessed for low energy availability using a newly developed, sport-specific questionnaire and clinical interview (SEAQ-I) (Keay, Francis, and Hind 2018). They found that 28 percent of the cyclists had low energy availability; five were thereafter diagnosed with an ED, and another five were found to have orthorexia. They found that 10 percent of these athletes had low testosterone and, despite prior supplementation, mean vitamin D level was low. Although training loads were positively associated with increased power-to-weight ratios as expected, body fat percentage was not significantly linked to performance. They also found that male cyclists with low long-term energy availability experienced adverse effects on bone and endocrine function as well as decreased cycling performance. The authors emphasized how this fact is in direct contrast with the riders expressed views, which are widely accepted in cycling circles and perpetuated by coaches, teammates, and cycling media, that achieving a low body weight and low body fat are important to cycling success. This misconception was seen as a precipitator for low energy intake and motivation for low body weight and leanness, and was also a factor in a cluster of underperforming cyclists who, despite high training volume, had low energy availability and thus lower than expected power-to-weight ratios and performance.

This research underpins the importance of debunking myths in sport about leanness and body weight being the supreme driver of performance. It highlights the importance of athletes fueling their bodies to reach their full potential and maintain optimal overall health.

Early Intervention Is Paramount to Long-Term Success

To prevent the many long-term adverse health effects associated with the female athlete triad, RED-S, and ED in athletes, early detection, diagnosis, and intervention is essential. It is worth repeating that successful treatment is also strongly correlated with establishing a trusting and multidisciplinary team that includes a physician, a registered dietitian well-versed in helping athletes with ED, and a mental health practitioner trained in ED to help the athlete deal with all aspects of the ED. Restoration of body weight is the primary goal and involves a combination of increasing nutritional intake and decreasing exercise expenditure that will also help to improve bone mineral density and normalize menstrual function (Mehta, Thompson, and Kling 2018).

Once the low energy availability has been addressed and corrected (to at least 45 kcal/kg/day [20 kcal/lb/day]) and weight gain has been achieved as necessary (to a body mass index of at least 18.5 kg/m^2 and at least 90 percent of ideal body weight), menstrual function in women should normalize and bone mineral density should improve (Mehta, Thompson, and Kling 2018). Restoration of weight should independently have a positive effect on bone loading and bone mineral density; however, in order to optimally improve bone health, normal hormone production will need to be assessed and restored as well.

Long-term complications for athletes with ED include many that will adversely affect both overall health and sport performance. Resulting amenorrhea, decreased bone mineral density, impaired cardiac function, and decreased immunity all adversely affect long-term health, while dehydration, impaired glycogen storage, decreased endurance, muscle weakness, psychological consequences (reduced mood, increased anxiety, and depression), and thoughts about food and body image or weight all have the potential to negatively affect performance across all athletes. A study conducted by Vanheest et al. in 2014 looked for performance effects of reduced energy availability and subsequent ovarian suppression in underfueling competitive female swimmers. As you are aware, a basic principle of training is to increase physical activity in order to elicit physiological adaptations, resulting in increased athletic performance. Not surprisingly, this study found a strong relationship between chronically low energy availability and an inability to appropriately adapt to training responses, leading to worsening performance. Athletes who have ED often have a misconception

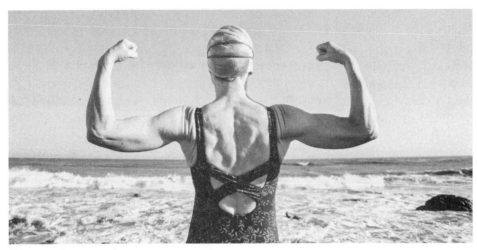

Recovery is strength.
Peathegee Inc/Getty Images

that an initial increased training load, restricted intake, and weight loss are going to improve performance. Long term, this simply is not true.

To further elucidate this critical point, we will now turn back to Ellen Hart, who bravely and honestly explains to us that athletes need to find their own personal motivations, something they value so much but that could be taken away from them if their ED continued to gain control. My hope is that this chapter, and Ellen's story, will help athletes recognize when they should seek the help they need and stick with the work it takes to gain full recovery from an ED.

A review article (Thein-Nissenbaum 2013) suggests that due to the compounding long-term adverse effects of ED in athletes, adults in their 30s and older should be screened for past history of the female athlete triad and assessed for current ED components at their routine physical examination, and appropriately treated or referred for help as needed. Since about 50 percent of peak bone mass is accrued during adolescence, history of ED during that time will predispose Masters athletes to low bone mineral density (BMD), osteoporosis, and increased risk of fractures. Adult women with AN and amenorrhea that began prior to age 18 have been shown to have lower BMD than those who developed amenorrhea after age 18, even after controlling for duration of amenorrhea. Even runners with "elevated dietary restraint" had significant incidence of lower BMD than runners without elevated restraint. This suggests that dietary restraint may itself be associated with negative consequences on long-term bone health even in the absence of disrupted menstrual function. It has been shown that the most important factor in counteracting this bone loss is an increase in energy intake combined with decreased exercise intake as necessary, which results in normalization of body weight. Nutritional considerations important in facilitating bone growth include adequate total calories as well as adequate (but not excessive) total protein, calcium, vitamin D, iron, zinc,

Spotlight on Ellen Hart (continued)

What is the truth about recovering from an ED?

The first thing that I always say is that this is not a chosen disease. The second thing I say is that it is a compulsive-addictive gene that, in my family, had manifested in my grandparents as alcoholism and then for me as an ED. It is not a choice! I can tell you these things now, sitting here speaking to you only a few days before my sixty-first birthday. But still somewhere inside me, I can't help but think it was my fault even though I know that is not true. I did a lot of public speaking for a while in Denver and at college campuses, and then of course there was the movie made about me in 1996, *Dying to Be Perfect: The Ellen Hart Peña Story.* That said, there was initially no way I wanted any of that to be public. I never wanted my children to know this about me because you don't want to tell anybody that you were binge-ing and making yourself vomit. This is not something you really like about yourself.

Back before anyone knew I had an ED, a running friend was interviewing me for a piece she was writing, and she asked me to speak about my ED. I was surprised, and asked, "What eating disorder?" She had been the team manager for a U.S. team I was on, and she just knew. At that time, I could not admit to it. One day soon after that, I was on a run and I suddenly had to stop to cry, because I finally saw myself in the third person. I went home and wrote a little article about my ED. Since I was in DC and my life was public, someone saw it and brought it to the attention of the *Washington Post*, and then it was in *People* magazine, and before I knew it, I was approached to do the movie.

Every step of the way I said no, no, no—I don't want to be the poster child for ED. But then I realized something. My guardian angel or the cosmos or God or the universe spoke to me and guided me and said, "Ellen, this is an important message, and you can let people know the message, that ED are a serious illness and that people can get help for this. That help is available, and recovery is possible." So in the end, I got to be the messenger at a time when not a lot of people were talking about ED. Per the letters I received, my story resonated with others who had to put on a pretty smile but had something "eating them" inside. Whether it was drugs or alcohol or food or whatever they used to deal with the emotional discomfort and the things they wanted to numb and the things they wanted to push away. The responses I got back right after the movie released were amazing. I would open a letter that said, "Your movie gave me hope. I have been sick for 15 years, and I am finally going to get help."

How did you find your reason to recover?

Parenthood was the catalyst for my recovery. As I mentioned earlier, I kept think-ing I could get a handle on it, and yet it just kept getting worse. It got pretty ugly. I always thought that if X or Y thing happened, *then* I would get better. Maybe when I got married it would get better—but that didn't happen. Then I wanted to get pregnant and we had issues with infertility, which was not a big surprise since my hormones and body had been stressed for 10 years due to my ED. When I did get pregnant, I was so happy. I mentioned to my OB/GYN that sometimes I threw up, and he said, "Yeah, everyone vomits during pregnancy, so don't worry about it."

> continued

> *continued*

Obviously, I didn't really tell him I was bulimic, and he didn't have any clue why I had mentioned my vomiting, but I was very worried I would hurt my baby. Then at six months pregnant, I thought I was having contractions and that my baby would not make it. If I wanted anything in this world, I wanted to have children and be a good mother. So then I asked, or made a deal with the universe—or karma or whatever is out there: If I promised to stop bingeing and purging for three months until this baby was born, will you please give me a healthy baby? For the next three months it was really hard and uncomfortable because I didn't know what it was like to have food in my stomach or how it felt to let it digest. But in the end, those three months gave me the tiniest hold on being healthy. And after my perfect, beautiful baby was born, it suddenly didn't matter as much to me how quickly I ran or what size clothing I wore because there was a bigger purpose. I just wanted to be a good mom. That was a big shift for me. I was healthy for 11 years and felt like I was finally living again. I didn't have to have my head in the toilet or obsess about what I was eating or how much I weighed. It was an amazing liberation.

Then the healthier I got, the more our marriage fell apart. I suppose now that was predictable. I had always said, "Don't worry about me. I don't need anything. I don't need communication or love or intimacy" because I had my ED. And of course none of this was articulable back then, but as I got better I realized what I wanted and needed. We had a downward spiral until we decided to separate and divorce.

How has your journey been?

There have been a few times I have slipped back into old bad habits. The first time, I had been healthy for so long and didn't realize I could go back to my ED, but looking back on it, I guess it makes sense: I was in emotional distress again, and I fell back into the ED. I instinctively turned back to the thinking that had held my emotional distress at bay in the past. I wanted to be better and to be able to keep my children, and so I went to a 12-step program and to therapy, and now I have been healthy again for 17 years.

There was also one time when I came in second at a race and some stupid human being actually said to me, "Well, you know why you got second. Just look at the woman who got first—she is 10 pounds lighter than you," and that triggered me for a bit again. I actually said to him, "Don't joke about that. I have a history of an eating disorder." But it was too late; what he said stuck for a while. And he should have known better than to say something like that to someone, but he didn't. No one should ever say anything like that to anyone.

I will say that I am 97 percent healthy, and it is something that I am incredibly grateful for. It doesn't mean that all struggles have been eradicated, but at this point, I want to nourish my body in healthy ways. Now, even if I eat more than my body needs for a day—either emotionally or just fun eating—it is not like the old days where it becomes a whirlwind in which I have to eat everything really fast and totally out of control. Now it is just that I ate more that day, more of the foods that I really like.

Ellen's Favorite Postrace Meal

Usually, I want scrambled eggs and a bread item. Then shortly after that, I seem to want fruits and vegetables, especially after a long race, where you have gone a good portion of the day eating really simple carbs. I just want that fresh taste.

and vitamin K. Additionally, supplemental calcium is generally recommended at 1,000 to 1,500 milligrams daily along with 600 to 1,000 IU of vitamin D.

Decreased calorie and protein intake in athletes with ED also leads to decreased protein synthesis and increased muscle breakdown (for energy) when inadequate intake is available, which has far-reaching performance implications as well as possible life-threatening cardiovascular complications. Bradycardia (resting heart rate less than 60 beats/min) and hypotension are seen across all ED and have been said to be useful as an initial marker of an ED, especially in athletes (Sardar et al. 2015). It is important to note that these symptoms generally improve once eating behavior has been normalized.

Underfueling and low energy availability contribute to impaired mood and increased rates of anxiety or depression. Thein-Nissenbaum (2013) points to increased rates of suicide and suicide attempts of up to 10 to 20 percent in individuals with AN and up to 25 to 35 percent in individuals with BN. The prevalence of concurrent mood disorders warrants referral and treatment, whether it is a stand-alone diagnosis or as a result of the presence of an ED.

Finally, it is critical for us all to remember that ED recovery is a lifelong quest, something to never be taken for granted. In telling her story, Ellen Hart explained the commitment necessary for ED recovery.

Bottom Line of Eating Disorders in Masters Athletes

Underfueling and the continuum of ED and disordered eating affect Masters athletes of all abilities and across most sports. Nutritional interventions such as increasing food intake to an adequate level and normalizing eating patterns are paramount to both long-term recovery and athletic performance. A multidisciplinary team including medical, nutritional, and psychological support can benefit athletes as they work through the complexities of symptoms, complications, and comorbidities associated with ED and long-term underfueling or malnutrition. Adequate fueling and weight restoration can lead to slowing or reversal of many of the consequences of ED including lowered BMD, mood disturbance, and cardiac changes, and can improve overall health and athletic performance.

On the next spread, we will hear from Stephanie Roth Goldberg, an athlete and sports psychotherapist whose knowledge and wisdom about treating ED will shed additional light on the intricacies of identifying, working through, and overcoming an ED in athletes.

Spotlight on Stephanie Roth Goldberg

Stephanie Roth Goldberg, LCSW, is an ED and sports psychotherapist in New York City, an endurance athlete, and mom of two. She is a certified eating disorder specialist who holds a certification in intuitive eating, training in cognitive behavioral therapy, and much more. I have been fortunate enough to collaborate with Stephanie on many cases of athletes with ED over the years, and I value her knowledge and her way of thinking about food, fueling, exercise, and our bodies.

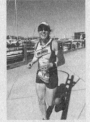

© Stephanie Roth Goldberg

What are the dangers of long-term ED you see in Masters athletes?

The longer you are underfueled, the more likely your bone density is going to decrease. Also, restrictive and eating disordered athletes will tell me that they see their heart rate getting lower and they think they are getting fitter—but there definitely comes a point at which they are breaking down and their critically low heart rate is rapidly becoming a medical issue.

How can athletes decide whether their motivation to exercise is healthy or not?

I ask my athletes struggling with overexercising to do a three-minute body scan to see how they are really feeling, then decide whether they should train today. More training is not always better. It is just your anxiety that says, "I need this run in order to complete my marathon in a month." It is not based in reality. *Guilt* is a key word I use with athletes and should never be a reason to exercise. Is guilt going to help you cross the finish line? No! We want to examine what is fueling the desire to work out or to choose to eat or skip a food. If you are unsure, make a pros and cons list (you can do this quickly in your head), then make an empowered decision. Is it an ED thought or a healthy thought? If you check in, find that your body feels fine, and know that you will actually feel better if you run, then go out and train today. But if it is tied to food, as in, "I think I should exercise because I ate a cupcake," that is another thing entirely. The key here is divorcing your training plan or exercise from food. If I am craving a cupcake, that has nothing to do with whether I have moved or not. My taste buds are not connected to my muscles; I am not honoring my body and my senses and my thoughts if I am tying my desire to eat with my desire to move.

What are some ED red flags people should look out for?

Refusing to eat out is always a big red flag. It shows distrust that our bodies can handle a normal amount of oil—or whatever the fear is around the food. This too goes in the anxiety bucket—and it goes toward the restriction of socializing, which is another aspect of our health. Another red flag is comparing your training and nutrition plan to someone else's. This competitiveness or hyperawareness of what others are eating or doing—doing another workout because someone else is doing it or not eating when you know you should because no one else is—shifts us away from focusing on what our bodies need. Turning inward and listening to our bodies is how we will truly be successful. Inflexibility around food is also a red flag. Say you are at a party where the cake looks delicious and you still refuse to eat it. You deprive yourself the enjoyment of eating that cake based on a preconceived notion regarding your need to exercise or the number of calories you "should" take in. Food rules as identity is another red flag. It is not true that good athletes do not eat cake. Nor is it true that if you want to be a good athlete you cannot eat cake. Avoiding cake (or dessert, carbs, or any food or food group) should not be part of your athlete identity. Those of us who work in the field of athletes with ED hear the generalizations and pressures within the community of elite athletes, which can be so hard. As we see all too often, there are groups of people who think it is normal or even noble to have not eaten sugar for 20 years. Let us tell you, that is neither necessary nor noble. Finally, if you are surrounded by people who are all in this disordered mentality, it becomes hard to know what is normal. The checks and balances are off, and it speaks to why it is important to have a good sports dietitian and psychotherapist involved directly with the coaches and athletes to encourage athletes to be in tune with their bodies.

Can you speak to those who may be experiencing binge eating?

All the research shows that bingeing happens when we restrict. BED often follows a period of restriction. If someone is afraid that once they start eating something they are not going to be able to stop, it is likely because they are in a restrictive cycle with their food in general or that specific type of food. The only way to work on this is to "legalize" the food and eat it in a way in which you enjoy it, and trust that once you allow yourself to eat the foods you like and you connect with your body, you are not going to binge. If you are connected with your body, the likelihood of bingeing is greatly decreased.

How do you go about helping athletes recover from an ED?

I challenge my clients to take a month or more in the off-season to really work through the anxiety around eating more and resting more. We might begin with something such as eating breakfast on a nontraining day. We talk through their anxiety about doing this and see that it is OK. Then they see they can run a mile as fast, if not faster, or lift as much weight, if not more weight, when they fuel their body properly. Then they start to realize that eating less was not helping them and that they are feeling and performing better. They think about food less and can concentrate more at their day job. They begin to trust and listen to their body.

Can exercise and fueling serve as either positive additions or negatives in our lives?

Yes! Exercise and competitive athletics should contribute to you being more of you, not make you less of you. The key question here is, "How can I think about my training or exercise as contributing more (better mood, more energy, more pride, increased strength, more community if I am with a group, more fun) rather than less (less weight, less energy, less enjoyment, less fun)?" When you restrict food, it is hard to think about expanding other aspects of your life such as careers, interests, and relationships. It really affects every aspect of your life. This is certainly a case in which more is not always better; all the research shows that even a 10-minute walk decreases anxiety and depression. But if you are too focused on getting all of your miles and training sessions in, then you have removed the benefit of anxiety reduction and made exercise anxiety-producing.

Stephanie's Favorite Postrace Meal

After a triathlon or marathon, I usually want a burger and fries, or if the race ends early, it is bacon, egg, and cheese on a bagel. I also like to have a bag of candy from Dylan's Candy Bar.

Resources for Information and Screening

If you believe that you or someone you know is exhibiting signs or symptoms of an ED or disordered eating and an unhealthy relationship with food and body image, there are plenty of ways to seek help. I have provided a list of resources, places you can go to find more information, and screening tools. Initial screening tools are widely available and can be used to start the conversation and help you decide whether to seek referral for formal evaluation and diagnosis. Once you suspect a problem, it is always advisable to consult with a medical professional for a physical examination, a mental health professional, and a sports dietitian who specializes in working with athletes with ED.

• The **National Eating Disorders Association (NEDA)** website has a free, short interactive screening tool (www.nationaleatingdisorders.org/screening-tool) that can be used as an initial self-assessment to screen for risk or presence of an ED.

• The **Female Athlete Screening Tool (FAST)**, available since 2001, screens for ED and atypical exercise and eating patterns in athletes. The tool is available at uhs.nd.edu/assets/165496/female_athlete_screening _tool_2011_12.pdf.

• The **Female Athlete Triad Screening Questionnaire** is a free resource at www.health4performance.co.uk/wp-content/uploads/2018/09/Female-Athlete-Triad-Pre-participation-Evaluation.pdf.

• **EAT-26** (www.psychology-tools.com/test/eat-26) is a widely used first-step screening tool that can be used to gauge initial risk and help determine when one should consult a qualified professional for further assessment and diagnosis.

• **Sport Specific Questionnaire and Clinical Interview (SEAQ-I)** (Keay, Francis, and Hind 2018) is available at https://www.ncbi.nlm.nih.gov/pmc/articles/PMC6196965/bin/bmjsem-2018-000424supp001.pdf.

• The **Exercise Dependence Scale (EXDS)** (Hausenblas and Downs 2002) at www.personal.psu.edu/dsd11/EDS/EDS21Manual.pdf is a 21-question screening tool that asks you to honestly answer questions about your feelings about and need to exercise.

• The **Eating Disorder Examination Questionnaire (EDE-Q6)** at www.corc.uk.net/media/1273/ede-q_quesionnaire.pdf can be printed out and completed at home. It screens for eating disorder behaviors over the past 28 days.

Although these tools are available online, I cannot stress enough that studies have shown that whenever possible, these questionnaires should not simply be handed to athletes to complete and return. They are much more effective at eliciting true and honest answers when administered by an interviewer who can observe the athlete's movements and facial expressions as they answer each question.

These websites include useful information on eating disorders:

- AN: www.nationaleatingdisorders.org/learn/by-eating-disorder/anorexia
- BN: www.nationaleatingdisorders.org/learn/by-eating-disorder/bulimia
- BED: www.nationaleatingdisorders.org/learn/by-eating-disorder/bed

---

We will now begin part III on nutrient timing and fueling your training, games, and races. Chapter 11 covers how much and what you need to eat before your competition to ensure you are well fueled and ready to perform your best. Then, in chapter 12 we will move into race- and game-day fueling guidelines and examples. Finally, in chapter 13 we will discuss nutrition for recovery, a topic that Masters athletes in particular need to fully understand.

PART III | NUTRIENT TIMING

11 | Precompetition Fueling

Over 50 years' worth of research supports the notion that athletes who begin their competition after ingesting adequate pre-exercise fuel produce significantly better performance results than those who begin in a fasted state (Ormsbee, Bach, and Baur 2014). Fueling before a race, game, or training session will top off your glycogen stores (available energy storage), increase the insulin response from your pancreas, increase glucose uptake by your cells, and increase the glucose available for oxidation (use) in your working muscles. Studies point to increased insulin response and lower fat oxidation following pre-exercise carbohydrate ingestion, which can be perceived as negative until you carefully analyze the entire physiological and metabolic picture; then it becomes clear that performance is improved when carbohydrate is consumed. This performance increase is most apparent for exercise lasting longer than 90 minutes, when glycogen stores begin to become limited.

If you are an athlete who mistakenly thinks you can't or shouldn't fuel up before key training sessions or races, I am confident that after reading this chapter, you will find a way to help you to feel your best and fuel your performances. In case you are concerned about a possible decrease in blood glucose during exercise following carbohydrate ingestion, it is important to know that studies show near-baseline blood sugar readings when carbohydrate is consumed in recommended amounts (1-4 g/kg [0.5-2 g/lb] body weight one to four hours prior to commencing exercise) (Ormsbee, Bach, and Baur 2014).

Initial studies on this topic, performed in 1967, led to the recommendation of avoiding carbohydrate intake in the hour before exercise (Jeukendrup and Killer 2010) or eating low glycemic index carbohydrates during that time. Jeukendrup and Killer (2010) also reported that since the initial studies, many groups have studied this phenomenon using different carbohydrates, types of exercise, and timing of ingestion, demonstrating that although insulin concentrations will be high following carbohydrate ingestion, glucose uptake will be

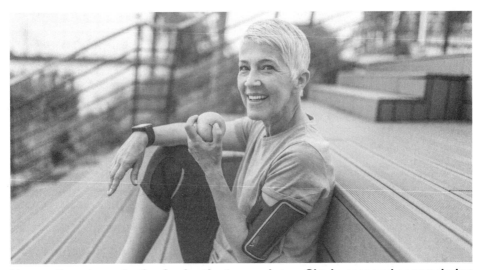

Use caution when selecting foods prior to exercise, as GI tolerance and energy during competition are most important at this time. Choose higher fiber foods, including apples and whole grains, only if they sit well with you.

dragana991/Getty Images

increased and glycolysis will also be stimulated. This cascade lasts for only 5 to 20 minutes and has not been shown to significantly affect glycogen use or exercise performance in a negative way. The overall conclusion is consistent; based on current research, ingestion of carbohydrate preceding exercise will improve performance.

Athletes who have experienced hypoglycemia or reactive hypoglycemia may want to ensure their pre-exercise carbohydrates are eaten more than one hour prior to commencement of exercise to minimize any transient dip in blood glucose. You may also want to experiment with including a small amount of protein with the precompetition meal and a brief warm-up immediately after fueling to help offset any potential rebound. You should then take in carbohydrate during your training and competition, which you will learn about in chapter 12. The bottom line is that consistent performance benefits are demonstrated in athletes who have adequate carbohydrate intake, so it is beneficial to prioritize a prerace or precompetition meal and to practice this often in training. The profiles later in this chapter will provide you with examples of what accomplished Masters athletes eat when they want to perform their best.

What to Eat

When asked about the best types of foods and carbohydrate to eat before a training session or competition, the mantra I repeat each time is to choose low-fat, low-fiber, moderate-protein carbs that you have eaten in practice and know settle well for you when you are nervous. See tables 11.1 and 11.2 for examples of pregame carbohydrate amounts and foods.

TABLE 11.1 Recommended Carbohydrate Intake Before Exercise

Time prior to exercise	Carbohydrate amount
30 minutes	Up to 0.5 g/kg (0.23 g/lb) (as tolerated)
1 hour	1 g/kg (0.5 g/lb)
2 hours	2 g/kg (0.9 g/lb)
3 hours	3g/kg (1.4 g/lb)
4 hours	4g/kg (1.8 g/lb)

TABLE 11.2 Pre-Exercise Carbohydrate Recommendations in Action for a 140-lb (64 kg) Athlete

Time prior to exercise	Food or beverage consumed
30 minutes	One banana OR 8 oz sport drink + one piece of toast
One hour	Two slices bread + 2 tbsp jam + 1-2 tbsp nut butter + half banana
Two hours	PB&J bagel sandwich (bagel + 2 tbsp jelly + 2 tbsp peanut butter) + one large banana + 1 cup sport drink (or 4 oz juice)
Three hours	4 x 4 inch pancakes with 2-3 tbsp maple syrup or honey + 1 banana + 1 cup milk of choice + 1 granola bar + 8 oz sport drink or 1 energy gel *
Four hours	Pasta meal (2-3 cups pasta + 1-1.5 cups tomato sauce + large ciabatta roll) + fruit smoothie (1 cup skim milk + 1 cup berries + one banana + 1/2 cup oats) + dessert (two cookies) **

* This can be spread out over the three hours prior to competition (e.g., pancake meal three hours prior, banana one hour later, and granola gar + sport drink approximately one hour prior to start time).

** This can be spaced out before competition as desired (e.g., pasta meal four hours prior, smoothie two hours prior, cookies with meal, or switch to an energy gel closer to start).

You may have already heard of the glycemic index (GI), which is the measure of the degree to which a carbohydrate food will produce a rise in blood sugar two hours after ingestion. The effects of high and low GI foods on subsequent athletic performance have been examined, with inconsistent results. Low GI foods (lentils, apples, yogurt, fructose, pasta, nuts) tend to have more fiber and more overall nutritional value, and are foods Masters athletes should consume on a regular basis for overall health benefits. Consuming them before exercise yields at least similar performance results as consuming high GI foods, and specific precompetition meal carbohydrate choices should be made on an individual basis based on GI tolerance and preference.

That said, most of us have had the unfortunate experience of eating too many low GI or high-fiber foods too close to practice, a competition, or a race, and having to spend the entire session dealing with abdominal cramping, gas, or diarrhea, and subsequently decreased performance. Therefore, a balance needs to be achieved between overall intake of low GI foods and leaning toward more high GI or lower-fiber, easier-to-digest foods (e.g., bread, potatoes, glucose) before key or intense workouts and leading up to competitions. High GI foods are also great choices for athletes with high total calorie and total carbohydrate needs as a way to take in more carbohydrate calories easily. Gastric emptying

TABLE 11.3 Low-Fiber Preworkout Carbohydrate Sources

Food	Portion size	Carbohydrate (grams)
Grains		
Bagel (plain, egg, salted)	1 large	60
Cereals (less than 2 g fiber per serving)	1 cup	25-35
Cream of wheat	2/3 cup, cooked	18
Bread (white)	One slice	15
Rice (white)	1/3 cup, cooked	15
Pasta (white)	1/3 cup, cooked	15
Waffle, pancake	One small (4" diameter)	15
Vegetables		
Potatoes, skinless	1 cup, cooked	30
Fruit and fruit juice		
Fruit juice, no pulp	1 cup	30
Cherries	10-12 cherries	15
Pineapple	3/4 cup	15
Banana	1 medium	30
Snacks		
Popsicle	One large	17
Crackers	Six small	15
Pretzels	3/4 oz	15
Rice cakes (white)	Two cakes (4" diameter)	15
Dairy products		
Chocolate milk	1 cup	27
Greek-style yogurt (flavored)	2/3 cup	16
Milk	1 cup	12

time (how long it takes a food or beverage to leave your stomach), fluid absorption rates, and gastrointestinal comfort are things that most athletes spend a good deal of time contemplating and experimenting with. Table 11.3 provides a list of easy-to-digest preworkout and precompetition choices.

On the following pages, you will hear from Stephen England, a marathoner and ultramarathoner who also has type 1 diabetes and an impressively optimistic outlook on managing a chronic disease.

What You Really Need to Know About Carbohydrate Loading

When completing workouts without glycogen depletion, normal restoration of glycogen stores can be seen within 24 hours as long as both decreased training volume and adequate refueling and carbohydrate intake are present

(Burke et al. 2011). As we discussed in chapter 5, the concept of carbohydrate loading (increasing carbohydrate storage in the muscle and liver using precompetition dietary and training manipulations) is one that was first used in the late 1960s and early 1970s (Bartlett, Hawley, and Morton 2015) and has continued to be widely studied ever since. This makes sense since we know that after about 90 minutes of exercise, we expect to see a 10 percent decrease in work power output or speed due to low available muscle glycogen. Current sport nutrition guidelines include specific carbohydrate reference ranges for the days and hours leading up to your competitions and stress the importance of practicing your race- or game-day fueling strategies during training.

In 1967 athletes commonly followed an initial carbohydrate loading protocol that involved a full six- or seven-day depletion and repletion in an effort to maximize muscle glycogen storage and therefore extend endurance capacity for events lasting longer than 90 minutes. This protocol called for a three-day, low-carbohydrate diet with high training volume followed by a three-day refeeding period wherein athletes would increase their carbohydrate intake to 8 to 12 grams of carbohydrate per kilogram (5-6 g/lb) of body weight per day (Bartlett, Hawley, and Morton 2015). Athletes profiled in this book who followed this early protocol say that it was difficult to follow and left their legs feeling heavy, but they followed it because that is what they were taught they were supposed to do and they wanted to run their best.

More recently, since the early 2000s, athletes have followed a much simpler method that entails 24 to 36 hours of rest combined with increased carbohydrate intake (8-12 g/kg [4-5 g/lb] of body weight/day). Thankfully, Bussau et al. (2002) demonstrated that trained athletes can achieve maximal muscle glycogen storage by combining one day of high carbohydrate intake (10 g/kg [5 g/lb] of body weight/day) along with one day of physical inactivity. This much more practical method is easier to implement and also works for frequently competing (weekly or biweekly) athletes who could not use the traditional carbo loading method nearly as often as they compete. Recent studies in Masters athletes support that more than 8 grams per kilogram (4 g/lb) of body weight per day of carbohydrate is adequate to induce carbohydrate loading in older athletes (Close et al. 2019). However, knowing these facts and achieving these high carbohydrate intake goals are often two different matters entirely.

The overall goal is to increase your carbohydrate intake to promote supercompensation (maximized storage above normal baseline levels), which in turn has been shown to increase endurance performance by 2 to 3 percent for races over a specified distance. This means that increasing your carbohydrate intake and stores could get you a 2 to 3 percent PR (Burke et al. 2011). Studies of professional cyclists doing multiple-day stage races such as the Tour de France, for whom daily endurance competition is the norm and for which carbohydrate loading is impossible, show the body's inability

Spotlight on Stephen England

Stephen England, who is 40 years old and originally from England, has called New York City home for the past 13 years. Stephen has been living with type 1 diabetes since age 14, and is a runner with Team Type 1 Elite (Type 1 Diabetes or DM1) and an ambassador for Team Novo Nordisk. He has run more than 80 marathons and ultramarathons in the United States and around the world, including a 2:45 personal record (PR) at the 2018 Boston Marathon, sub-24 hours at Western States 100-Mile Endurance Run, and 3 days and 3 hours (with just 3 hours of sleep!) at the inaugural Tahoe 200 Endurance Run. Stephen has completed every race he has started. His mantra is that if he can't quit diabetes, why would he ever quit a race? Stephen shares fueling strategies and life lessons as an endurance athlete with type 1 diabetes.

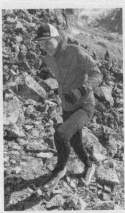

© Stephen England

What motivates you to run and to fuel well as a Masters athlete?

I really thrive off people who ask, "Why are you going to run 100-plus miles? Are you crazy?" It gives me more power to keep going. But really, I am motivated to eat well for three main reasons. The first is that I know how I perform on a training run when I eat badly, and I know how it feels to perform well when I fuel well, and I like the latter much better. The second reason is that I'm the first one in my family to really be an athlete. My third motivation is to help control my diabetes. With diabetes, exercising every day is so important for blood sugar control and overall health. Whether it's walking the dog or running an hour in the park, we need to move our bodies every single day. This is something we can do for ourselves and our health, but sadly, many people don't do it.

How does having DM1 affect your nutritional needs and intake?

Having type 1 diabetes for a long time has made me more conscious of what my body needs, which has actually served to make me a better athlete. The first thing that was obviously important when I was diagnosed was learning about carbohydrates and taking insulin; that kept me alive. The second most important thing in my diabetes life was getting a continuous glucose monitor (CGM) six years ago. The CGM is a small wearable device that tracks blood sugar every five minutes all day and night. Once I got a CGM, my world as an athlete opened up 10-fold. To be able to see my blood sugar on the fly and see the trends all the time is just mind-blowing. Now I couldn't live without it.

How has your nutrition intake changed as a Masters athlete?

My nutrition routine is fairly consistent but has morphed gradually over the years toward a higher quality level overall due to maturity. For example, I had been eating cereal, including Frosted Flakes, for years, and that evolved over the past 10 years into oatmeal or granola. I like thinking of myself as a car and the food as the gasoline. If I am constantly putting in really crappy, cheap gasoline (or not enough gasoline), then my car is going to run really badly (or not at all). I feel the difference in my body every year; everything is more of a challenge. I am very conscious that nutrition is integral in terms of continuing to be able to compete.

How do you fuel up for long runs and races?

I eat a very high-carbohydrate diet day in, day out, so I am always pretty well fueled. I still live by the whole "get a nice pasta meal before a race" mentality. But what has worked for me for the past few years is having my pasta meal at lunch. I know I am well fueled, I can sleep well, I can digest it, I can manage my blood sugar, and I can go to the bathroom in the morning before the race. About two hours before my race starts I eat about 65 grams of carbs' worth of oatmeal, plus a yogurt and half a banana. Since I have DM1, I have to count my carbohydrate intake every time I eat so that I can match my insulin to it. Of course, I then have to have the diabetes conversation in my head. Where is my blood sugar? Is it too low? (Normally not, but I need to check.) Is it too high? If so, I may have to take a bit more insulin to cover it. I am very conscious not to take too much insulin before a race, because the worst thing for me, or anyone with diabetes, is to go low. I can run when I'm a little too high, but even a little too low, and I'm really in a bad place. Once I am 10 minutes from the starting gun, if my blood glucose (BG) is not in the 150 to 180 range, I am already off to a bad start—so I can't let that happen. During races, I have my CGM set on vibrate to notify me if my BG is high or low.

How do you manage having type 1 diabetes (or any chronic disease) as an athlete?

When people get diagnosed with something like diabetes, they get scared, and they either change their life, they freak out, or they ignore it. If you have been diagnosed with DM1 or anything else, do not immediately jump into thinking that it will change your life in a negative way. Yes, you are going to need to look at your diet, and you are going to track your BG, but it is going to be OK. You can absolutely eat a high-carb diet and be an athlete and have diabetes; you just need to take appropriate insulin. I'm a proven case study on that. I can run 100 miles and eat a high-carb diet and be successful. People who say you can't are wrong. For me, it is just one more factor. As an athlete, you need to train well, fuel your body, have the right clothing, stick to a plan with a pace—you get the idea. There are multiple factors to having a great race day, and managing my diabetes is one more thing I must do. I check my BG every day regardless of my training. I live with it 24-7. I breathe it. I almost kind of thrive off it, if you can't tell. I enjoy being different now, and I enjoy having that one more factor to overcome.

Do you consider yourself a role model for athletes with DM1?

My teammate and I run the Boston Marathon every year, and we're obsessed with our PRs. Whether I run what I want or not, I post it on social media and about 500 people comment on it. Someone with a five-year-old with diabetes comments, my grandma comments, my mom comments, and very quickly I realize that it's not about the number or the time, it's about the story—that I live with type 1 diabetes and I can complete anything I want to. It quickly puts things into perspective and reminds me of the bigger picture.

Stephen's Favorite Postrace Meal

My postrace meal is always something savory. After all the gels, sport drinks, and cola I use to get me through a long race, I need a change. I seek out a vegan burger and fries alongside a local craft beer or two. I remind myself I deserve it!

to increase glycogen storage to greater than baseline (precompetition levels) with such intense carbohydrate usage. In such instances, athletes are advised to consume large enough quantities of total carbohydrate (see table 5.1) in both food and liquid supplement form in order to replace as much glycogen as possible between repeated competition days. See table 11.4 for a summary of your best carbohydrate fueling strategies.

TABLE 11.4 Pregame or Prerace Carbohydrate Needs

Fueling strategy	Recommendations
Pre-exercise	Take in 8-12 g carbohydrate/kg (3-5 g/lb) of body weight in the 24 hours prior to competition that lasts less than 90 minutes.
	Increase to 10-12 g carbohydrate/kg (4-5 g/lb) of body weight for the 36-48 hours prior to competition lasting more than 90 minutes.
	Take in 1-4 g carbohydrate/kg (0.5-2 g/lb) of body weight in the final one to four hours prior to competition to further increase body glycogen stores.
Fueling for second session	Refuel with 1-1.2 g/kg (0.5 g/lb) of body weight four times after exercise if less than eight hours before the next session.
Other considerations	Consume foods that are low fat, low fiber, and high carbohydrate. Consider including a source of protein.
Summary	Individualize and fine-tune your pretraining and precompetition fueling by identifying how your body responds to each of these recommendations. Remember that science gives us great places to start, but only you (and your coach or sports dietician) know how you respond to each nutritional or training manipulation.

Data from Burke et al. (2011).

On the next spread, you will hear from celebrated runner and author Roger Robinson. But first, let's examine what a prerace-day meal plan might look like for an endurance athlete.

Sample Prerace-Day Meal Plan

This sample prerace-day meal plan is designed for a 140-pound (64 kg) endurance athlete.

Day before the race

Breakfast (6:30 am)

- Four medium pancakes topped with 1 cup strawberries and 2 tablespoons maple syrup
- Two hard-boiled eggs
- Glass of orange juice

Short final training session (8:30 to 9:30 am)
Post-workout snack (10:00 am): Recovery smoothie with 8 ounces yogurt, one scoop protein powder, 1 cup tart cherries

Lunch (12:00 pm)

- One large flour tortilla, 1 cup white rice, 4 ounces tofu, avocado to taste
- Two large handfuls of pretzels
- Glass of lemonade (possibly with a pinch of salt)

Snack (3:00 pm)

- One can V8 juice + two servings of crackers + one banana
- Or one can V8 juice + one high-carb energy bar (e.g., Clif bar) + one banana

Dinner (6:00 pm)

- Large baked potato with 1 tablespoon butter
- 3 ounces chicken
- Two slices Italian bread
- Two cookies

Snack (8:30 pm)

- One bowl (1.5-2 cups) low-fiber cereal (e.g., Rice Krispies) with milk of choice
- Or other high-carb energy bar or bread

Race day

Breakfast

- One large bagel with peanut butter
- One banana
- 8 to 12 ounces sport drink of choice

Spotlight on Roger Robinson

In 70 years (so far) as a runner, Roger Robinson has represented both England and New Zealand in world championships and set marathon Masters records (in age groups 40+ and 50+) at Boston and New York. He is also one of running's most acclaimed authors, having written the best seller *When Running Made History*. Roger is an inspiration to all of us who aspire to continue to be active throughout our lives and to enjoy the runs, rides, swims, and games along the way.

What is your overall nutrition philosophy?

My philosophy has always been and increasingly is about balance. In life and particularly in nutrition, the more varied—and the less you do or eat the same one thing day after day—the better. I did some of my literature work on Darwin and the impact of evolution, and have always believed that we have survived due to our ability to adapt, so I eat different foods every day. When Kathrine* is away, I'll rotate what I cook; something with rice, then pasta, then potatoes, plus chicken or fish or a vegetarian meal. Then when I get bored with cooking, I'll go out for pizza. When we do go out, I often find the foods served don't taste natural. I don't want my food "all messed up" with extra sugar and salt all over everything, and I am certain that funny things happen to your body if you eat like that all the time.

* Roger's wife is Kathrine Switzer, a champion of both the women's running movement and now active aging movement, who appears in chapter 1.

Have you made any nutritional changes as a Masters athlete?

When I was growing up in wartime London, we couldn't afford to get enough to eat, and even the school meal they gave us was hardly adequate. Now I can afford to eat and drink more, which for many can be dangerous. One quite amusing consequence, which I am aware of so am conscious of avoiding it, is that I have this habit, almost compulsion, to eat everything on my plate, because I was brought up hearing, "Eat it up now because there might not be enough tomorrow." It still makes me feel a bit guilty to leave food on the plate, but I pretty much have that under control. Once I got beyond about 50, I couldn't run 100-plus-mile weeks anymore. My overall nutritional habits have not really changed, but my total intake has certainly decreased.

What's your advice on prerace nutrition?

I'll give you both my serious answer and my comical one. Before a race, my only real rule has always been to eat what I am used to. I don't want to give my body a surprise on race day, and I don't want to eat anything that might send me to the bathroom while racing. While I stick to what I know, not everyone always does, and since the history of running is full of nutritional follies, my bit of comical advice includes the following:

- Before your next marathon, no water for 24 hours beforehand or during the race.
- Oodles of apple butter the night before.
- One hour before, eat a two-inch thick steak.

- If it's hot, at 15 miles drink champagne.
- At 20 miles, eat a meal of fruit.

Or better, be thankful you are running in the first era to understand nutrition science and read the rest of this book for much better advice than mine!

While each of the above nutritional follies may sound ridiculous as you read them now, they all actually occurred and affected marathon history.

- In the 1908 Olympic marathon, Tom Longboat was closing in on the leaders when he was given champagne at mile 15 and dropped out two miles later.
- In the 1904 Olympic marathon, Felix Carvajal of Cuba looked like the likely winner at mile 20 until he stopped to eat a bowl of fruit, then suffered convulsive stomach cramps.
- In 1934 Jock Semple was one of the favorites to win the Boston Marathon but ate a 2-inch steak the hour before the start in an attempt to "fortify" himself, leading to crippling nausea on Commonwealth Avenue.
- In 1967 it was Amby Burfoot who lost his chance to win Boston by succumbing to a craving for apple butter the night before. He then spent much of the race making pit stops. (Luckily, he learned his lesson and came back to win the following year.)

In all seriousness, lacking sound sport nutrition knowledge, earlier ages took an approach to nutrition that was derived more from instinct than science. Water seemed weakening; steak seemed fortifying. Now we know better. In the marathon, water is strength. My best advice to all runners is this: Don't let yourself fall prey to mistaken beliefs about nutrition and let them undermine your next marathon effort!

You have been running for a long time. Do you have any other nutrition rituals?

After a race, our ritual, which in all honesty is *really* what makes it worth continuing to race into your 70s and now 80s, is that we go to a really gritty diner and get the ultimate American binge breakfast. This is our comical ritual, but the serious point is that food can and should be fun. These are foods we don't eat normally, and after a race we pretend this is what we crave because this is what we want—and we eat together and enjoy it. There is an element of comic reward.

In later life a lot of things get taken from you, like when I had to have both of my knees replaced and didn't think I'd ever run again. As I have gotten older, I have decreased my training and eaten less, but I also didn't want to make myself more miserable by following a spartan diet and denying myself foods I like. I didn't want to agonize over what I ate or feel guilty about it, and I didn't want to be miserable, so I didn't and I still don't. I also believe in comic pragmatism. More balance + less stress = feeling happier overall.

Roger's Favorite Postrace Meal

Rack of lamb with six veggies or the aforementioned greasy diner breakfast.

Modified Starches and the Masters Athlete

No pre-exercise fueling conversation would be complete without a discussion and review of modified starches. High molecular weight (HMW) starches are thermally modified starches that are modified to be either heavier and more slowly digested than traditional carbohydrate sources such as maltodextrin, or lighter than and therefore more rapidly digested than maltodextrin. When taken before exercise, using slowly digestible HMW modified starches such as UCAN in place of lower molecular weight (LMW) starches has been shown to decrease insulin response and increase fat oxidation. However, these changes have not translated to significant performance improvements in subsequent time trial performance (Ormsbee, Bach, and Baur 2014).

HMW modified starches with a high GI and fast digestion rate such as Vitargo have been studied for potential effects on exercise performance following previous glycogen-depleting exercise. Studies suggest that the consumption of 100 grams of these modified starches in the two hours following glycogen-depleting exercise may improve subsequent time trial performance by 10 percent, possibly due to greater glycogen resynthesis between exercise bouts (Oliver et al. 2016). These findings warrant further research in a wider range of athletes but may be particularly interesting to those athletes engaging in repeated bouts of high-intensity exercise throughout the day and who have traditionally had difficulty replacing muscle glycogen between sessions.

As athletes, we should read the scientific literature on nutrition, then test out nutritional strategies in practice. We need to listen to what our body, brain, and gut are telling us and adjust until we feel our best. (Roger Robinson, in the previous sidebar, is a good example of this. A Masters record holder, he balances common-sense fueling with comedic pragmatism.) I see too many athletes consume the same foods before multiple training sessions and races with the same undesirable effects (e.g., indigestion, cramping, bloating, and fullness or bowel urgency) before they realize that strategy is just not working for them. Just prior to key training sessions and competitions is a time to throw away your preconceived notions of what you *should* be eating and which foods are *best* or *healthiest*, and listen to what your body is telling you.

Fueling Up With Protein

The addition of a protein source to the pre-exercise meal has been shown to be beneficial for athletes concerned about any possible negative effects due to increased insulin response produced by pre-exercise carbohydrate intake. This is generally easy to include because most carbohydrate sources contain some protein. Studies have shown that adequate overall and pre-exercise protein intake becomes even more paramount in instances of low carbohydrate availability and restricted energy intake (Thomas, Erdman, and Burke 2016). Such protein intake may also help support muscle glycogen resynthesis and enhance muscle protein synthesis when consumed just prior to strength and endurance exercises alike.

Adding protein to your pre-exercise carbohydrate intake seems to increase the body's natural glycemic response compared to carbohydrate taken alone, though more research is needed to establish true connections as well as optimal protein types and amounts. Specifically, the amino acids arginine, leucine, and phenylalanine have been shown to stimulate the pancreas, help increase glycogen synthesis, and promote glycogen sparing during exercise (Ormsbee, Bach, and Baur 2014). They may also increase postexercise glycogen resynthesis. For this reason, it is worth trying to include 8 to 10 grams of protein with your pretraining and precompetition meal. This can easily be accomplished by eating one egg, 4 ounces of Greek-style yogurt, 3 ounces of tofu, or 1 to 2 ounces of chicken along with carbohydrate, or may be obtained directly from your carbohydrate sources depending on your prerace food selections. This may be of special consideration to ultraendurance athletes seeking to enhance recovery from prolonged and muscularly exhaustive exercise.

One of the best ways we can continue to get the most out of our training sessions and maximize our performance is to ensure that we take in adequate fuel daily. While our daily carbohydrate needs as athletes will vary by sport, intensity of exercise, and stage of our lives, we as athletes should periodically assess our carbohydrate needs throughout the years to ensure we are continually meeting our potential.

We will continue our discussion on optimal fueling as we move into chapter 12, where you will find practical intake advice based on timing and duration of activity as well as real stories from more athletes.

12 | Competition-Day Fueling

Throughout this book, you have learned about the importance of carbohydrate, protein, and fat for Masters athletes to promote longevity in sport. You read about the changing fluid needs of Masters athletes and ways to ensure you are well-hydrated for each workout, game, race, and competition. I covered supplements to consider and did a deep dive into what to do to ensure you are eating enough and to learn to recognize the signs and symptoms of low energy availability in sport and disordered eating in Masters athletes. You learned how to fuel up for competition day. Now we will put it all together as I show you how to fuel for your best race or game day ever.

No longer do nutrition and hydration recommendations differ simply by sport, but by the challenges each athlete must fuel up for and recover from on any given day. Endurance athletes need to fuel with lots of carbs but also need more protein than previously was thought to be the case. Team sport athletes also benefit greatly from following a nutrition and hydration plan on game day, especially for multiple-day competitions or multiple-game days. And while it is true that resistance training (RT) athletes need adequate protein for muscle repair and growth, they also benefit from adequate carbohydrate and fluid. In this chapter, I highlight the importance of carbohydrate, protein, fluid, and salt consumption on competition day performance, show examples of practical fueling for different athletes, and leave you with a much better understanding of *your* individual race-day fueling needs.

Carbohydrate Needs During Competition

In the 1960s scientists first realized that muscle glycogen was a key and limiting factor in exercise performance. By the 1980s studies had shown that a mere 22 grams of carbohydrate per hour (88 calories' worth), helped boost performance when taken during exercise, so a 6 to 8 percent carbohydrate solution (sport drink) taken every hour was recommended. Next, early and more consistent carbohydrate intake was shown to further improve performance (Kerksick et al. 2017), and the recommendation shifted to advising carbohydrate intake every 15 minutes throughout activity. Since then, studies have shown improvements in not only endurance athletes, but also improved mental drive, agility, dribbling accuracy, shot accuracy, and decreased fatigue in team sport athletes and performance benefits in RT athletes (Kerksick et al. 2017) when carbohydrate is ingested before and during competition. If you had read up on your game-day fueling needs anytime from the 1990s through 2004, you likely would have read the recommendation that athletes should aim to ingest 30 to 60 grams of carbohydrate per hour during exercise, an intake range still quoted online, in magazines, and among athletes and coaches. However, this recommendation was based on research showing that absorption rates for glucose peaked at 1.0 gram per minute (60 g/hr) regardless of body size, age, or sport (Jeukendrup 2014).

Newer science shows we can and should train our guts to take in more. By 2004 new studies showed that it is possible for athletes to absorb more than 60 grams of total carbohydrate per hour during exercise when multiple transport carbs are ingested. This has been backed up by subsequent research (Ormsbee, Bach, and Baur 2014) and is very exciting news, because the more we can take in and absorb, the longer and faster we can go. Since fructose is absorbed by different transporters than glucose, ingestion of both carbohydrate energy sources leads to an absorption rate of 1.5 grams of carbohydrate per minute during exercise (up to 90 g/hr) (Jeukendrup 2014). This is a 50 percent increase in what was previously thought to be a maximum absorption rate. Once we train our guts to accept this higher carb intake, we can reap the benefits, including lower rating of perceived effort (RPE), better maintenance of cycling cadence, and reduced fatigue.

As exciting as that revolution was in the world of sport nutrition, a new study (Viribay et al. 2020) demonstrated an ability for elite ultra runners to take in and absorb even higher amounts of total carbohydrate per hour, up to 120 grams of total carbohydrate per hour (2 g/min). They cite anecdotal reports of this high carbohydrate intake in elite cyclists, some marathoners, and Ironman triathletes after training their guts in practice, and their study showed promising results in terms of decreased RPE and better recovery with this higher carbohydrate intake during competition.

Carbohydrate intake can serve to help athletes maintain pace, motor skills, concentration, and RPE as well as to spare muscle glycogen by providing substrate for the body to burn as fuel, preventing drops in blood pressure and

Maximum Carbohydrate Intake During Exercise

Your carbohydrate intake needs and absorption rates during exercise do not depend on your age, gender, training status, or body weight, and these intake guidelines should be implemented by all athletes looking to perform their best and recover efficiently (Jeukendrup 2014). This helps explain why we don't see too many 7-foot-tall, 220-pound Olympic marathon runners—it takes more energy and carbohydrate to move a larger individual gracefully and swiftly over 26.2 miles, but they cannot take in (or benefit from) any more total carbohydrate than a smaller runner. Regardless of whether you are 5' tall or 6'7", and whether you weigh 120 pounds or 220 pounds, try to train your mind and gut to take in 60 to 90 grams of carbohydrate per hour.

---

activating the central nervous system (CNS) reward centers. Regardless of sport, athletes whose competition lasts more than 60 minutes and who will be working at greater than 65 to 70 percent $\dot{V}O_2$max will not only be racing against their competition but also against depleting glycogen stores. This is where sport drinks and chews, gels, and even real food can be beneficial during races and events.

Additional research has shown that as athletes become dehydrated, reliance on carbohydrate stores for energy only increases (Kerksick et al. 2017), which is yet another reason for athletes who race and compete in the heat to ensure they stay on top of meeting their carbohydrate needs on race or game day.

Carbohydrate need is further amplified for those athletes competing early in the morning (after sleeping and thus an overnight fast), because studies have shown that beginning fueling early during such circumstances can help offset *some* of the performance decreases seen and expected when fueling is limited or inadequate. If feel you cannot take in the amounts recommended for your precompetition fuel to optimize your performance on the day of, please continue to practice taking in more, but also begin fueling early and often during your competitions.

In a 2002 study, Kimber et al. found that athletes competing in the Ironman (IM) Triathlon (2.4-mile [3.9 km] swim, 112-mile [180 km] bike ride, and 26.2-mile [42 km] run) demonstrated an average intake of 1.0 gram of carbohydrate per kilogram (0.4 g/kg) of body weight (women) and 1.1 gram per kilogram (0.5 g/kg) of body weight (men). Not surprisingly, they noted that athletes tended to take in carbs at a higher rate while cycling (1.5 g/kg [0.7 g/kg] of body weight/hr) versus while running (Jeukendrup 2014). (As I have noted through this book, sports dietitians do not recommend carbohydrate intake based on grams per kilogram of body weight in athletes, because carbohydrate absorption rates are not dependent on body weight, but this is how it was reported in the article.) Their study demonstrated that 120-pound (54 kg) triathletes took in an average of 55 to 60 grams of carbohydrate per hour overall throughout the entire competition, with about

80 grams per hour being taken in during the bike portion. Meanwhile, triathletes weighing 160 pounds (73 kg) took in an average of 73 to 80 grams of carbohydrate per hour overall over the entire bike and run segments of the event, and 109 grams per hour on the bike. While this study seems to suggest that larger triathletes took in more calories from carbohydrate per hour during their Ironman event, an important reminder again is that fueling during events should not be based solely on body weight, as maximum absorption rates are gut dependent rather than body weight dependent. All athletes, regardless of height or weight, should aim to maximize their intake within the above recommended guidelines to maximize their performance. Ultimately, IM endurance athletes, whose events last anywhere from 8 hours (for professionals) to 16 or 17 hours for some participants, should understand their need for carbohydrate fueling during such a long and grueling event.

Let's start by looking at endurance athletes, especially those training for long-course races such as triathletes racing for 70.3 or 140.6 miles in one day, marathoners, and ultramarathoners. These dedicated athletes tend to rise early and fuel often—and with good reason. They often swim, bike, run, and fuel for hours on end in both training and on race day. I remember reading a book before I completed my first Ironman (140.6) race in Lake Placid back in 2001, and the first thing that struck me was that *every* Ironman athlete profiled in the book seemed to get up at five o'clock in the morning and start eating right away. This is not a coincidence! Long-course endurance athletes (runners, triathletes, cyclists, and swimmers) often begin their race day with a full breakfast such as bagel with eggs or with peanut butter and banana, coffee, and a sport drink before they arrive at the race venue. That is generally followed up with another energy bar, gel, or banana and water about 15 minutes prior to the time they jump into the water or begin the grueling multihour competition. Most long-course triathletes that I have met, either personally or professionally, over the past 20 years of my both participating and helping athletes fuel for this event, call nutrition the fourth leg of triathlon. We simply cannot swim, bike, and run for 8 to 17 hours straight without carbs, fluid, and sodium to keep our body moving forward and our brain functioning enough to push us to do so. Most endurance athletes know they need to begin experimenting months before their race to learn what sits well for them and to train their guts.

What I find generally surprises almost everyone, from first-time racers to elite pros and Olympians, is just how much they can and should take in during these races. I generally help athletes calculate their sweat rates and then design a fluid and carb intake plan according to their taste preferences, tolerance, and racing needs. As endurance athletes, triathletes, marathoners, and others should always train to take in at least 60 grams of carbs per hour and possibly up to 90 grams as tolerated and depending on race-day temperature. We practice drinking different sport drinks on the bike and run, often testing out what will be served on the course, to ensure each athlete can tolerate that formula or learn they need to carry their own. Throughout a three- to six-month training cycle leading up to such an event, we pack peanut butter and jelly (PB&J) sandwiches, energy bars, gels, energy chews, dried fruit, rice balls, waffles, and even salted boiled potatoes in our bike jerseys, running shorts, and fuel belts, and test out which foods, types of carbs, and flavors continually sit well and taste good to each athlete. We practice getting into good recovery nutrition habits, because how an athlete recovers from one training day, training block, or early-season race will determine how strong she continues to feel in later training sessions and peak races later in the season.

Let's look at what a race-day nutrition plan might look like for a long-course triathlete.

Sample Race-Day Fueling Plan

This sample race-day fueling plan was designed for a 120-pound (54 kg) long-course triathlete.

Prerace fuel

Breakfast (5:00 a.m.)

- Two frozen waffles with syrup
- Two eggs
- One banana

12 to 16 ounces sport drink sipped throughout the morning and one or two cups coffee as desired

One energy gel packet and 4 to 6 ounces water around 6:50 am

During-race fuel (7:00 a.m. wave start)

On the bike

- One 20-ounce bottle of sport drink per hour (about 35 g carbs/hr)
- One third to one half carbohydrate-based energy bar every 30 minutes (about 30 to 45 g carbs/hr) or equivalent in rice balls, PB&J sandwiches, salted potatoes, etc.
- Water to match sweat rate and minimize weight loss to less than 2 percent during event
- Salt tablets as needed to match sodium loss needs in sweat (about every 30-60 min)

On the run

- 4 to 6 ounces sport drink every 15 minutes (28-42 g carbs/hr)
- One energy gel every 30 minutes (about 40 g carbs/hr) or equivalent in energy chews
- Water as needed to replace sweat loss and minimize weight loss to less than 2 percent

(continued)

Sample Race-Day Fueling Plan *(continued)*

- Salt tablets as needed to replace salt lost in sweat (about every 30-60 min)
- Other items from race volunteers or special needs bags: crackers, sandwiches, even Snickers bars

Postrace fuel

ASAP (less than 30 minutes after finishing) consume 22 to 40 grams of protein plus 45 to 60 grams of high glycemic index (GI) carbs in food or recovery drink (e.g., recovery shake with 25 to 40 g of protein, one banana, 8 to 12 oz milk [low-fat cow's milk or oat milk], or food if able to tolerate it right away)

Postrace meal 1 (consume within one to two hours after recovery drink) that contains 45 to 60 grams of carbs and 22 to 40 grams of protein (e.g., a sandwich with 4-6 oz tuna or steak, 1 cup fruit, 1/2 to 1 cup bean and corn salad)

Snack (about two hours later) that contains 45 to 60 grams of carbs and 20 to 30 grams of protein (e.g., large piece of fruit, 6-8 oz Greek-style yogurt; or oat- or grain-based granola, thick slice of pumpkin or banana bread, or muffin and 6-8 oz Greek-style yogurt)

Dinner (if you are still awake two hours after your snack) that consists of a balanced meal with 45 to at least 60 grams carbs, about 30 grams of protein, good fat, and veggies (e.g., 2 cups cooked pasta with tomato sauce or olive oil, 4 oz chicken or tofu, salad with avocado and olives, bread)

Bedtime snack that includes casein protein (from milk, yogurt, or supplement) if optimal recovery is imperative (i.e., another match, key workout, or race is within 24-48 hours), or enjoy any treat you wish

Reasons to Optimize Carbohydrate Intake and Train Your Gut

Recent research has demonstrated that overall dietary intake may play an important role in determining how much carbohydrate an individual athlete is able to absorb on race or game day. For those of us who have been competing in or participating in endurance sports for decades, we can still remember a time when we did not think we could ingest anywhere near what we now routinely take in during long rides, runs, and races, and we now know that the gut is in fact trainable. (In the next chapter, on recovery, you will read that ultra runner and coach Ramon Bermo initially thought I was crazy when I explained his carbohydrate needs to him, and I can assure he is not the only athlete to ever say that to me.) You can train your gut by ensuring you take in adequate total carbohydrate in your daily life and by gradually increasing the amount of carbohydrate you take in during your training sessions and eventually your competitions. Taking in carbohydrate is inherently easier for cyclists than runners (or during the cycling leg versus the run leg for triathletes) due to logistics as well as gastrointestinal tolerance. Intake during competition can also be tricky for skill-based sports during which athletes have access to fluid and carbohydrates only during breaks in the game such as halftime. The bottom line is that whatever your sport, it behooves you to find a way to meet your needs; your performance depends on it. See table 12.1 to help you decide where and how to begin better fueling your best performances.

Adding Protein

Studies have shown promising results for many types of athletes when protein is consumed, along with carbohydrate, during training and racing (Kerksick et al. 2017). Coingestion of these two important macronutrients has been shown to increase muscle protein synthesis during a two-hour RT session and may also be helpful for athletes engaging in ultraendurance exercise (Thomas, Erdman, and Burke 2016). Studies have shown that even during a 40-minute RT session, adding protein plus carbohydrate ingestion can lead to a 49 percent decrease in muscle glycogen lost and improved long-term training results even if no performance benefit was measurable during that training session or competition (Kerksick et al. 2017). Other research has demonstrated that during three hours of cycling at 45 to 75 percent $\dot{V}O_2$max,

TABLE 12.1   Optimal Fueling for Masters Athletes .

Duration of competition	Exercise intensity	Fueling recommendations	Other notes and strategies
<45-60 min	<75% $\dot{V}O_2$max	Water is often adequate.	Consider trying carbohydrate mouth rinsing for competition lasting 30-60 min. Consider additional fueling if extremely intense or important session.
45-75 min	High intensity; >75% $\dot{V}O_2$max	Begin to take in some carbohydrate to maximize performance.	Consider sport drinks and other rapidly absorbable carbohydrate sources.
1-2 hr	Any intensity, but especially if >75% $\dot{V}O_2$max	30 g of carbohydrate/hr.	Use mostly sport drinks plus some gels or energy chews.
2-3 hr	Any	Aim for up to 60 g of carbohydrate/hr.	Practice fueling in training to test palatability and gut tolerance.
>2.5-3 hr	Any	Experiment with taking 60-90 g up to 120 g of carbohydrate/hr.	Include multiple carb sources (glucose/maltodextrin + fructose) for absorption of >60 g/hr. Higher carb intake is associated with improved performance, better recovery, and lower RPE during prolonged competition. Add protein, up to 0.25 gm/kg/hr (0.11 g/lb/hr).

Data from Thomas et al. (2016); Byrje et al. (2011); Jeukendrup (2014); Viribay et al. (2020).

ingestion of carbohydrate plus protein improved endurance and decreased muscle damage. In a two-hour RT session, 0.15 grams of carbs plus protein taken just prior to and every 15 minutes during the training session led to increased muscle protein synthesis, decreased muscle protein breakdown, and a net overall increase in muscle accrued (Kerksick et al. 2017). Whether your goal is to optimize your performance today or your long-term recovery for improved muscular or endurance performance, it makes sense to fuel your body well during your competitions.

Mouth Rinsing

As strange as this might sound, recent research has demonstrated that simply rinsing your mouth with a carbohydrate solution can improve time trial performance during short-duration exercise lasting about one hour (Baltazar-Martins and Del Coso 2019). Carbohydrate rinsing, as it is often called, appears to activate receptors on the tongue and in the CNS that lead to increased performance and has been shown to decrease the time to complete a course on a bicycle trainer and to increase cycling power (Baltazar-Martins and Del Coso 2019). Interestingly, and certainly a topic for further study, researchers noted a downside to mouth rinsing in higher reported RPE in the mouth-rinsing athletes. It should be noted that the performance advantage might be small for all but the fastest of athletes, and some studies have not demonstrated any performance effect with mouth rinsing, especially when testing athletes in a fed state (i.e., they had eaten a meal prior to the trial).

Athletes engaging in RT, power, and strength sports have traditionally recognized their higher needs for protein than the average inactive or less active person but often sell themselves short in terms of reaching their full potential by not fully embracing their carbohydrate (energy) needs. As we have discussed throughout this book, strength athletes do require carbohydrate to fuel their movements, brain, coordination, and mood. These competitors would be best served to include both protein and complex carbs in their precompetition breakfast and to follow that up with some essential amino acids (EAA) plus carbohydrate just prior to their event. Especially for those athletes who will be working hard for one and a half to two hours, sipping on a traditional sport drink with 6 to 8 percent carbohydrate (*not* sugar free) and that possibly contains EAA during their event will serve to help decrease muscle protein breakdown and increase muscle protein synthesis (Kerksick et al. 2017). Postcompetition nutrition will ensure each athlete recovers optimally and is ready to train or compete again sooner. Here's what a competition-day fueling plan might be for an RT athlete.

Sample Competition-Day Fueling Plan

This sample competition-day fueling plan was designed for a 180-pound (82 kg) RT athlete.

Breakfast (8:00 a.m.)

- Two eggs
- Two slices whole grain toast with butter or peanut butter
- Half avocado
- One bowl of fruit

Precompetition snack (2 hours before event; about 10:00 a.m.)

6 to 10 grams EAA or 25 to 40 grams total protein and 35 g carbohydrate (e.g., 5 oz chicken, one medium potato, or fruit smoothie with EAA powder)

Fuel during competition (12:00-2:00 p.m.)

Water or mouth rinse if competition lasts less than one hour, or sport drink as able 6 percent carbohydrate sport drink, about 4 ounces every 15 minutes if competition lasts one and a half to two hours

Fuel after competition

ASAP (less than 30 min after finishing) consume 25 to 40 grams of protein plus 35 to 65 grams of high-GI carbs in food or recovery drink (e.g., recovery shake with 25-40 g of protein, 1 cup berries, 8-12 oz low-fat cow's milk or oat milk)

Snack about two hours later (e.g., 3 oz of turkey jerky, one large fruit, 1 handful of nuts)

Dinner of a balanced meal with 25 to 40 grams of protein, carbs, good fat, veggies (e.g., 4-6 oz broiled fish, rice and beans, sautéed collard greens)

Bedtime snack of 8 to 12 ounces of low-fat milk and fruit or two cookies

For more on fueling, see the sidebar on the next spread about Olympic swimmer BJ (Bedford) Miller. She also explains how she navigated body image pressures at the elite level.

Spotlight on BJ (Bedford) Miller

BJ (Bedford) Miller is an Olympic champion and former world record holder in swimming; she and her teammates won gold for the United States in the 4 × 100 meter medley relay at the Sydney Games in 2000. BJ and I spoke about fueling as an elite and Olympic athlete and how she navigated the pressures of nutritional fads and body image while spending years of her young adult life in a bathing suit. She may just inspire you to love yourself a bit more than you ever have before.

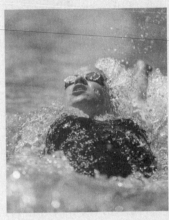

Al Bello /Allsport

What was your fueling like as an elite-level swimmer?

It may surprise some people to hear that I ate a bowl of Frosted Mini-Wheats every day before practice. People might say that wasn't a very healthy choice, but even when I lived at the Olympic Training Center, I ate them every day. I knew I didn't want to swim feeling too full, but I also didn't want to swim without having fueled my body. It was more about getting the calories in and less about paying attention to what nutritional buckets I was filling; it was just one insatiable bucket that I was constantly trying to fill. Many people don't realize that swimmers are classically overtrained. We trained for seven to eight hours a day, and my longest race was two minutes. It's nuts. Again, for that part of my life, it was all about getting the calories in. If it didn't move off my plate before I could stab it, it was going in my mouth, and that was it. This also disproves the myth that you can't swim within a half hour of eating. We did it every day.

How did you think about fueling for race days?

We swam and raced often, and needed something that was going to digest easily, so we ate pasta all the time—and it did provide us with the energy we needed. When you ask me now, I realize I was always more carbohydrate focused, even though I wasn't thinking in those terms back then. I was thinking about what my body was going to be able to process quickly, because I didn't want anything sitting in my gut when the gun went off. I needed to know I would feel comfortable racing, wanted to feel light and be able to race, and feel like I could attack at any time. I was always eating, always snacking. At meets everyone was constantly talking about carbo loading, which basically meant we were eating pasta or carbs and snacking all day long between races. We knew what it takes to really fuel such heavy training and performance, and we followed that.

How do you think the swimming culture affected your body image?

I was in a swimsuit for most of my life, so there's nothing you can hide. What was ironic was that despite the heavy training and need for a lot of eating, you still had this pervasive concept that everybody was fat. Even the skinniest person on our swim team would look at herself in the mirror and say, "Oh my God, my thighs look big!" And I'd think, "If your thighs look big, I'm a heifer." It was so bizarre. There was this conversation undergirding everything—not that it stopped us from eating, because we were working so much we had to. Fortunately, I didn't ever have an eating disorder, but on every team I was on since high school, there were always one or two girls that were really struggling with one. That part was pretty rough.

What nutritional changes have you made as a Masters athlete?

I can remember back to when I was training heavily, ordering pizza and getting mad if someone would take a slice. I would think, "This is my pizza. I train for six to eight hours per day and ordered all the things that I want on my pizza, so you can go get you own pizza if you want some." I would sit down and eat an entire freaking pizza, and think, "Ah, this tastes so good!" Of course, I wouldn't do it before practice. Now my volume of food intake has decreased as I train a lot less. I eat two pieces of pizza and I'm pretty full. I don't want a whole pizza anymore. I weigh a bit more than I did when I competed in the Olympics, but I am pretty stable here and pretty comfortable. I think if we are honest, we'd all love to lose 5, 10, or 20 pounds, but I know how hard it is to maintain that, and I am not really interested in how hard that is. So, I'm just going to chill up here. (*Author's note:* I could barely contain my excitement at this point in the interview at how cool BJ has managed to stay in regards to her eating and body image. What I wouldn't give to share that love of self with all athletes with whom I work.)

How did you get to such an amazing place, being happy with yourself and your body?

To be really honest with you, I was not in that great of a place leading up to competing in the Olympic Games. Up until then, I had felt like the answer to everything was getting to the Olympics. If I can just get there, then I'm going to be an Olympian for the rest of my life and everything is going to be better. I knew logically that wasn't true, but I thought maybe it would be for me. I guess I had to get to the mountain-top to prove that none of it was real, that I had made it all up. There is that brass ring mentality where you think, *Maybe if I just reach a little further it will be mine*, but at the same time, it propagates the whole mentality that the thing you want is outside of yourself, and it's not. It never is. Everybody's road is different. Mine had to lead to the Olympics until I could finally stand back and realize that nothing else changed. I'm so grateful for having had the experience, because it brought me so much peace and the realization that I can choose to be happy. That is really what our body perception is about and where nutrition plays into this too. A lot of the time, athletes think that if they control what they eat, they are going to look and perform a certain way, but this feeds into that unhealthy mentality. We need to have these conversations with and among athletes, and turn them around into thinking more healthfully and truly honoring our bodies for what they can do. We need to get to the point of saying, "I am going to really nourish my body in the right way."

BJ's Favorite Postrace Meal

If I had another race that day or weekend, it was usually more carbs, such as more pasta—something quick and easy that would turn into fuel for my next races. When I was finished swimming for the meet, I'd have a burger or an entire pizza!

Prerace Hydration

As we discussed at length in chapter 9 on fluids and hydration, beginning a competition in an underhydrated state may adversely affect performance for a wide range of athletes (Thomas, Erdman, and Burke 2016). Athletes can avoid this unnecessary situation by consuming 5 to 10 milliliters per kilogram of body weight (9-18 oz for a 120-pound athlete, 12-24 oz for a 160-pound athlete, and 15-30 oz for a 200-pound athlete) in the two to four hours before beginning their competition, and then continuing to drink throughout their event (Thomas, Erdman, and Burke 2016). Including some sodium in your pregame and during-game fluids may help promote better fluid retention and is generally encouraged for athletes competing in hot or humid environments, for at least 60 minutes, wearing heavy equipment, or excessively sweating.

Due to the wide range of sweat rates and sodium content of sweat between and among athletes and across a season, fluid intake guidelines need to be individualized to meet each athlete's specific fluid and electrolyte needs. Athletes sweat an average of anywhere from 0.3 to 2.4 liters (10-84 oz) per hour of exercise, so one-size-fits-all hydration guidelines clearly will not work. See table 12.2 for a review of your fluid needs during exercise.

Remember that Masters athletes should pay closer attention to signs and symptoms of dehydration, because age-related decreases in perception of thirst make it more likely that athletes will not realize they are becoming dehydrated (Thomas, Erdman, and Burke 2016). Also, as discussed in chapter 9, while many muscle cramps may actually be the result of muscular fatigue, they could also be the result of hypohydration and imbalances in

TABLE 12.2   Fluid Needs During Exercise

Hydration goal	Guidelines	Additional considerations
Replace fluid lost to sweat during exercise to minimize dehydration to <2% body weight	Most athletes will lose 0.3-0.8 L (10-27 oz) of fluid per hour due to sweat. Some athletes lose up to 2.4 L (82 oz) of fluid per hour.	Sweat rates vary widely among athletes and for individual athletes throughout the season and depending on acclimatization. Customize your fluid replacement plan based on sweat rate testing.
Minimize risk of hyponatremia	Do not consume fluids in excess of loss through sweat.	Include sodium (sport drink or other source) if you are a salty sweater, sweat more than 1.2 L (42 oz) per hour, are training or competing for more than 2 hours, or are exercising in a hot environment.
Increase (or decrease) as needed	Consider your individual sweat rate, climate, and acclimatization.	Sweat rate testing will help you determine the correct fluid replacement plan for you.

electrolytes. Athletes with such symptoms should be assessed for sweat rate and sodium or electrolyte content of sweat as able, and all athletes who are known to have high sweat rates or high sodium or electrolyte content of their sweat should be educated and monitored more closely to prevent resulting muscle cramping (Thomas, Erdman, and Burke 2016).

Each athlete will have his or her own unique struggles in terms of carrying, maintaining access to, and drinking adequate fluids (and sodium) during completion. As you might know from personal experience, or can easily imagine, it is difficult to drink while running a marathon at record-breaking pace, when spending a large percentage of the game time on the soccer field, or when trying to hold a line in a cycling time trial. Each of these needs to be practiced early and often during training so that your performance does not suffer due to an inability to reach for or take in fluids. For example, runners learn to pinch the cups handed to them by race volunteers in order to get a higher percentage of that fluid into their mouths rather than on their shoes or the athlete behind them. Cyclists and triathletes need to be confident in their bike handling skills in order to confidently and safely drink from their bottle attached to their bike. Team sport athletes, tennis players, and other such athletes need coaches, sports dietitians, and teammates who advocate for ready access to personalized fluid bottles during quick breaks and changeovers and for athlete rotations that allow for time to gulp down much-needed fluids, carbs, and electrolytes during long games and matches. The more all athletes and coaches learn and understand just how important adequate fluid intake and hydration are for athletes across all sports, the more these essential practices will be embraced by all involved in sport, and the better we will all feel and perform because of it.

Multievent and Multiday Competition Fueling

For athletes who will have multiple races, games, or competitions in a 24- to 48-hour period, game-day nutrition plays an important role in performance in subsequent events. The International Society of Sports Nutrition (ISSN) position stand on nutrient timing (Kerksick et al. 2017) states the importance of nutrition for optimal recovery when rapid repletion is needed and races or games occur with minimal time to recover and refuel in between. It stresses that when athletes have less than four hours to recover between events (training or competition), they should take in 1.2 grams of carbohydrate per kilogram (0.5 g/lb) of body weight per hour and eat or drink high GI (rapidly absorbed) carbohydrate. They also suggest that consuming 3 to 8 milligrams of caffeine per kilogram (1-4 mg/lb) of body weight and 0.2 to 0.4 grams of protein per kilogram (0.1-0.2 g/lb) of body weight per hour would be beneficial. Of course, these principles apply not only on competition day, but also to those athletes training multiple times per day and looking to maximize their recovery and long-term training and performance. For athletes who have the luxury of slightly more than 24 hours between competition bouts (or even between consecutive training days with intense or interval sessions lasting 85-90 minutes), consuming a total of 8 grams of carbohydrate per kilogram (4 g/lb) of body weight per day has been shown to be adequate to help athletes in sports such as soccer, basketball, hockey, and rugby to fully replete their glycogen stores so they're ready to play again (Kerksick et al. 2017).

Masters athletes in team sports have their own fueling challenges, especially during competition. Running to the sidelines to listen to coaches' midgame advice, discuss strategy, and gulp down several sips of a sport drink containing carbohydrate and sodium takes practice. Having a friend, teammate, or coach remind and encourage athletes to drink helps, as does having one member of the team already know and practice optimal game-day hydration and fueling; their example can have a trickle-down effect to other players. Any 6 to 8 percent carbohydrate sport drink is better than none or plain water for team sport athletes who need to perform their best throughout the entire game. Having energy bars, granola bars, fresh or dried fruits, and salted pretzels readily available for athletes to grab in locker rooms and on the bench can make the difference between winning or losing the game in the final minutes. We will now look at an example of what optimal fueling might look like for a team sport athlete during a weekend tournament.

Sample Competition-Weekend Fueling Plan

This sample competition-weekend fueling plan was designed for a 160-pound (73 kg) team sport athlete.

Breakfast upon awaking (about 7:00 a.m.)

- One large bowl of cold, ready-to-eat cereal or hot cereal with milk of choice
- One banana
- 1/4 cup granola
- 8 to 16 ounces water

Pregame 1 fuel (about 8:30 a.m.)

One scoop of protein powder (25 g of protein) mixed with almond or oat milk

Fuel during game 1 (9:30-11:30 a.m.)

Intake goal of 30 to 60 grams of carbohydrate per hour

- 16 ounces of sport drink per hour (32 oz total during a two-hour game)
- Two or three energy chews as able whenever off the field or court (ideally three or four total)
- One banana as tolerated at halftime
- 20 to 40 ounces plain water (per athlete's individual sweat rate needs)

Postgame 1 fuel (about noon)

ASAP, less than 30 minutes after finishing, consume 25 to 40 grams of protein plus 80 to 90 grams of high GI carbs in food or recovery drink (e.g., sandwich with 4 oz turkey, three handfuls salted pretzels, two pickles, one fruit, one cup coffee, water to replace that lost due to sweat [ideally using sweat rates])

Snack (1 p.m.), 25-30 grams of protein and up to 110 grams of carbs as tolerated (e.g., smoothie made with two cups fruit, 8 oz Greek yogurt or a scoop of protein powder and ice plus any carbohydrate of choice [e.g., bagel or muffin] or 1-2 cups cooked pasta, 4 oz chicken or tofu, one cup orange juice, 8 to 16 ounces of water)

Pregame 2 fuel (2 to 3 p.m.)

Sip on sport drink as tolerated to goal fluid intake of amount lost due to sweat in game 1 plus 12 ounces

Fuel during game 2 (3:30-5:30 p.m.)

Intake goal of 30 to 60 grams of carbohydrate per hour

- 16 ounces of sport drink per hour (32 oz total during the two-hour game)
- Two or three pieces dried fruit as able when off the field or court
- One carb-based energy bar as tolerated at halftime
- 20 to 40 ounces plain water (per athlete's individual sweat rate needs)

Postgame recovery

ASAP consume 25 to 40 grams of protein plus 60 to 80 grams of high GI carbs in food or recovery drink

Dinner consists of a balanced meal with good sources of carbohydrate, protein, and fat (e.g., large burrito with rice, beans, meat of choice or tofu crumble, cheese, guacamole, and veggies, and water to replace sweat losses)

Bedtime snack includes casein from milk, yogurt, or supplement (e.g., 1 cup yogurt, 1 cup fruit, chopped nuts, and shaved chocolate, or shake with one scoop casein protein powder, 1 cup milk of choice, fruit, and ice) or any dessert desired

Carbohydrate and Protein for Recovery

As we have seen throughout this book, more studies are needed on Masters athletes and optimal recovery nutrition, but it seems that conflicting study results are likely due to the fact that Masters athletes, especially those ages 59 to 76 years, need more protein (possibly up to 40 g) to elicit the desired effects seen in younger athletes (Kerksick et al. 2017). In practical terms, your carbohydrate portion should generally be two to three times larger than your protein portion for your posttraining and postcompletion meal, snack, or shake. See table 12.3 for what that might mean for you based on your current body weight.

These guidelines should be helpful to athletes who have multiple races per day or back-to-back competition days, and especially for any athlete who for any reason has had inadequate prior total carbohydrate intake. Following

TABLE 12.3 Carbohydrate and Protein Needs Between Events and After Competitions

Nutrition needs between games, races, or matches	120 pound (54 kg) athlete	160 pound (73 kg) athlete	200 pound (91 kg) athlete
1.2 g of carbohydrate/kg (0.5 g/lb) of body weight/hour	65 g	87 g	109 g
OR 0.5-0.6 g of carbohydrate/kg (0.2-0.3 g/lb) of body weight every 30 minutes for 4 hours or until next meal	27-33 g every 30 minutes	36-44 g every 30 minutes	45-55 g every 30 minutes
0.2-0.4 g of protein/kg of body weight (0.1-0.2 g/lb) per hour	11-22 g	15-29 g	18-36 g
3-8 mg of caffeine/kg (1-4 mg/lb) of body weight	160-430 mg	218-580 mg	270-700 mg

these recommendations has been shown to help decrease muscle damage, promote euglycemia (normal or stable blood sugar), and increase glycogen resynthesis. Consuming carbohydrate plus protein within 30 minutes after completing your competition will help you replace your glycogen stores up to 50 percent faster than if you waited (accidentally or purposefully) more than two hours to do so. This is important because decreased glycogen stores have been shown to limit our ability to maintain our desired work intensity and leads to increased tissue breakdown, neither of which are desirable outcomes when our goal is to continue to perform (Kerksick et al. 2017). Again, this is true for endurance athletes as well as for RT, strength, and team sport athletes.

We will now turn to another inspiring athlete, Olympic medalist and marathon record holder, Deena Kastor, who exemplifies that listening to your body is always the best fueling and performance plan.

Spotlight on Deena Kastor

Deena Michelle Kastor is an accomplished marathoner, half-marathoner, road racer, and author of the book *Let Your Mind Run: A Memoir of Thinking My Way To Victory*. She won a bronze medal in the 2004 Olympics in Athens, Greece, won the Chicago Marathon in 2005, and the London Marathon in 2006 in a U.S. marathon record time of 2:19.36. Deena also won the women's Olympic marathon trials in 2008 and came in sixth in the 2012 Olympic marathon trials after having her daughter, Piper. She holds U.S. records on the road at the 8-, 10-, and 15-kilometer distances. As a Masters runner, Deena set the women's half-marathon record (1:11.38) in 2014 and again later that year (1:09.39). She also broke the women's Masters marathon record by more than one minute in Chicago in 2015, when at age 41, she ran 2:27.47. I am grateful to Deena for speaking to me, and for being a testament to the fact that athletes need to listen to and fuel their bodies well in order to maintain peak performance and optimal overall health.

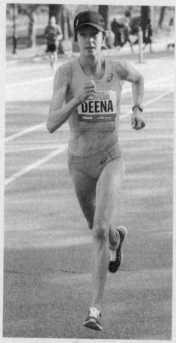

Brad Barket/Getty Images

How has your fueling changed over your career as an elite and Masters athlete?

Early on I would basically just throw stuff on a plate and not even heat it up. Then I realized I deserved better and decided that I would take five minutes to put the ingredients together and heat them up. Even today, if my daughter, Piper, and my husband are out, and I am eating by myself, I deserve to eat food that looks and tastes good. I will use spices, put a garnish on the plate, make a nice burrito—and it resonates on a deeper level. My overall goal is high quality: eating high-quality foods, getting high-quality sleep, doing high-quality workouts, and being with high-quality people. All foods are good foods, and I never denied myself anything I love. I would, and still, go into the kitchen and make a batch of delicious homemade cookies and enjoy them. I think we need to pay attention to how we feel after we eat certain foods or even how we feel when we eat with certain people. If you are eating your son's birthday cake and you are eating it with joy and surrounded by friends and family and thinking about a great year ahead, then you will enjoy the cake. But if you are eating the cake with a sense of guilt or because other people are watching you and it is stressful to you, then I think your body can tell the difference.

Have you ever felt you had to micromanage your nutritional intake as an elite athlete?

I have never counted calories or monitored my food intake, and always just ate by hunger, but during the build-up to the 2004 Olympic Games in Athens I saw

> *continued*

> *continued*

the sports dietitian at the IOC. They wanted to make sure I was getting enough of everything: calories, protein, carbs, fat, etc. She had me keep a food log for a week and told me I was eating 7,000 calories per day. Back then, when my mileage was really high, I craved sugar all the time. Whether it was in the form of cake or even some wine, I felt that I needed the carbs, calories, and energy, so I ate it. I know other elite athletes who really restricted their diet during training, but I never did. I understood that I did not need to and that it would not help me be a better runner or a healthier person if I did. I have seen a few anomalies of elite athletes who have had a restrictive diet and still manage to perform amazingly well, but more often, when I see other athletes who restrict calories and food groups or their overall intake, they seem to be injured more often and their careers are not as long. They are not thinking about their overall or long-term health.

What do you typically eat the night before a big race?

I typically look for a pesto pasta with salmon, or pizza with prosciutto and arugula on it. But I could also eat rice with some protein. I want to top off my carbohydrate stores plus protein for muscle and brain function. I know that the prerace dinner is a ceremonial meal, meaning I view it the same way I do my bib number—whether it is pizza or rice for dinner or bib number 2 versus number 5, whatever I have becomes my lucky meal and number for that day.

What is your marathon race-day fueling strategy?

I like to be up at least three hours before my race, which might mean four o'clock in the morning! I immediately chug a jug of water to hydrate my cells within every muscle. Then I go straight into making my breakfast, which is most often some type of nut butter on a few pieces of toast. Or I might put butter on my toast with some scrambled eggs and possibly a strip of fatty, salty bacon because, as I tell myself, marathon running is a fat-burning event, and I am sure the salt must help with the electrolytes I will need down the road. I also drink one or two cups of coffee, depending on the size of the cup. Then, until race time, I will continually sip on carbohydrate fluid. I will train with one brand of sport drink for a training cycle and let my gut get used to it, but luckily, they all sit pretty well with me. During

Gender Differences in Race-Day Fueling and Recovery

More studies are needed specifically in female athletes, who may need higher total carbohydrate and calorie intake to elicit the same response studies have shown in men (Kerksick et al. 2017). Some of this discrepancy may be due to physiological differences between the sexes, and another may be attributable to the fact that muscle protein synthesis will not be optimized unless overall nutritional needs are met and energy balance is achieved. It the race, I drink 4 to 6 ounces of fluid every 5 kilometers. I am constantly thinking about the tangent (i.e., the straightest line and thus shortest distance on the road course), where and when my next bottle will be, navigating the course correctly, and ensuring I am on pace. In training I make the drink slightly stronger than the directions say, minimally so, but so that I can get in a few extra calories. In addition to that, at 25 and 35 kilometers I take 4 to 6 ounces of water with JetBlack GU in it. I significantly feel the boost of the caffeine and the extra calories. There were times in my first few marathons when I started to feel depleted, so I added extra calories ahead of those times in the race so that I was never bonking.

Have you had any nutritional mishaps or fueling fails?

In 2002 I tried a drink with protein on a long run, and after 12 to 14 ounces I was so thirsty, felt my stomach getting bloated, and felt a dehydration headache. Then when I finished, I puked up everything, so that experiment was done. Another time, when I had giardia and lost 6 pounds, I was acutely aware that I needed to put that weight back on quickly. While I will usually have tea and a scone for my afternoon snack, at that time I started making milkshakes with peanut butter, protein powder, and a banana in order to get the weight back on.

Do you have any final words of nutritional wisdom to share with us?

When you choose to eat beautiful, delicious foods and listen to your hunger, you get the same feeling that you get with a runner's high—a feeling of satisfaction and of rewarding yourself. I want to make choices that are good for my running and are also good for my overall health, my family, and for me as a mother, because being a mother is the most important thing in the world to me. The way I see it, if I am making choices that are supposed to be good for my running performance, then they should also align with my overall health. If I was not eating enough and not giving my body what it needs, then is it really good for my overall health? No, it can't be. Is it good for my family? Also no. It is so important to have your checks and balances.

Deena's Favorite Postrace Meal

I love pizza, but most of all, wherever I am, I like going to a great place for something very ethnic or spicy, and when I come home, I crave a good burrito.

makes sense that athletes who are not consuming adequate total calories regularly will not reap the same benefits from even well-planned nutrition for before, during, and after competition, and studies need to ensure athletes are indeed in energy balance when investigating such hypothesis.

Throughout this chapter we have discussed the science behind optimal race-day nutrition and practical strategies for fueling your next competition. I provided several examples of what your next competition-day fueling might look like with much-needed carbs and protein. We examined ways endurance, strength training, and team sports athletes can practice meeting their during-race or -competition fueling (carbs and protein) and fluid (water and sodium) needs. I gave you some tried and true examples you may already be familiar with, such as bottles filled with sport drink during marathons or at halftime and bananas between sets, as well as some crazier-sounding ideas including stuffing your cycling jersey pocket with boiled, salted potatoes and eating PB&J sandwiches while sweating profusely and breathing heavily. Whatever your hesitation or concern is regarding increasing your intake of carbs, protein, fluid, or sodium before, during, or after your events, I guarantee you can work through it and fuel your body for both better short-term performance and improved longevity in sport.

In the next chapter, we move on to the final piece of the sport nutrition puzzle: nutrition for optimum recovery.

13 | Recovery Nutrition

I have saved one of the most important aspects of sport nutrition for last in this book: nutrition for recovery. As we continue to pursue athletic goals into our 40s, 50s, 60s, and beyond, the importance of replacing what we burn during training and racing, repairing our muscles and maintaining our muscle mass is essential to our longevity in sport, continued performance, and overall health.

I never want to see an athlete miss out on proper recovery from her latest training session or competition because she didn't have the time or hadn't realized it was *that* important, so I will address some common concerns. Early-morning exercisers (like me) will see by the end of this chapter that it is worth either getting up a few minutes earlier or preparing something the night before in order to ensure you give your body what it needs in between completing your workout and hurrying back out the door for work. Evening exercisers will understand why it's important to prepare or pick up food before you return home sweaty and tired at night or come up with another creative strategy to ensure you never go to bed hungry and underrecovered again.

More and more of us are seeking to maintain fitness and strength as we navigate life and athletics throughout our long lives. The average age of the finishers of the Hawai'i Ironman World Championship in Kona is 43 years old, and Masters athletes now comprise approximately 50 percent of all finishers in that grueling 140.6 mile race in the heat (Gray 2019). These athletes are prime examples of successful aging by maintaining a high level of sport performance throughout their lives. Thankfully, as more of us continue to strive to push boundaries in terms of fitness and performance through the decades, more research is being done on Masters athletes, which is finally illuminating the fact that our needs are likely greater than those of our younger selves or counterparts, especially when it comes to recovery.

Most Masters athletes are familiar with the need to alter their training plans as they advance in age (i.e., fewer high-intensity days, more rest or easy recovery days, fewer competition days) and assume that a loss of muscle mass and metabolic rate is inevitable. Recent research highlights that by paying attention to our increasing needs for recovery nutrition, we can extend our athletic lives and overall fitness for much longer than was previously thought.

You may recall from when we previously discussed protein needs as Masters athletes in chapter 6 that the recommended daily allowance (RDA) for protein for the general population is only 0.8 grams of protein per kilogram (0.4 g/lb) of body weight per day. This equates to a mere 44 grams of protein a day for a 120-pound (54 kg) athlete, 58 grams for a 160-pound (73 kg) athlete, and 73 grams for a 200-pound (91 kg) athlete. However, as we also discussed in detail in chapter 6, daily protein needs are higher for Masters athletes, both in general and following exercise. In this chapter we will delve deeper into what your postworkout and overall protein needs are for optimal recovery.

We have also already discussed overall daily carbohydrate needs (chapter 5), as well as preworkout and -competition fueling (chapters 11 and 12). Now, we put them all together to see how each piece of your nutritional intake puzzle contributes to your muscle repair, glycogen repletion, and overall recovery. After this final chapter, you will be armed with all the knowledge you need to fuel your body optimally for your best record-breaking self at all ages.

Current State of Nutrition for Masters Athletes

Recent reports show, and my personal work with a wide range of Masters athletes supports, that only one third of U.S. adults over age 50 are meeting the RDA for daily protein (Louis et al. 2019), which means that an overwhelming two thirds of our over-50 population are behind in protein even before their increased needs as athletes. They also reported that Masters triathletes tend to consume less total energy (calories) after exercise than their younger counterparts and less total carbohydrate (only 0.7 g/kg [0.3 g/lb] body mass) versus what is recommended for optimal recovery (1.0 g/kg [0.5 g/lb] body mass) and less than their younger counterparts (1.1 g/kg [0.5 g/lb] body weight). However, Masters athletes' needs are at least the same for total carbohydrate intake and higher for total protein.

The bottom line is that inadequate total energy intake and inadequate macronutrient intake during the recovery period immediately after exercise, a race, or a game will impede your recovery in many ways.

The silver lining is that studies and my own professional experience show that Masters athletes are able to maintain a higher training volume when their overall nutritional intake is adequate to meet their overall energy needs

(Louis et al. 2019). Eating enough overall has also been shown to help maintain resting metabolic rate (RMR), increase overall metabolism, and lead to a more favorable body composition. We will get into the specifics on what you need to recover and perform at your best, but first, see the sidebar on the next page for an account from Paul Thompson, an energetic athlete who has been both a runner and coach for decades.

Carbohydrates Are Still King

The more we train, the more work our bodies need to do to replenish muscle and liver glycogen (carbohydrate energy) daily as well as repair and grow muscle proteins before we train or race again. These important physiological processes naturally require substrate, namely carbohydrate and protein. Early work in this area supported the fact that adequate carbohydrate intake after exercise is imperative for athletes who need to continue to repair their bodies and maintain a high level of performance throughout a session or lifetime. This is because as glycogen levels decrease, our ability to do work also declines, as does our ability to maintain our desired exercise intensity or work output (Kerksick et al. 2017). As if that wasn't enough reason to get excited about how far recovery nutrition can take us, rates of tissue breakdown have also been shown to be higher without adequate intake of both carbohydrate and total energy. As such, restocking muscle glycogen is considered a primary goal for all athletes following training and racing. And it should make intuitive sense that protein intake after exercise is important, especially when muscle-damaging exercise has occurred or when gains in muscle size and strength are desired.

When I began my career as a sports dietitian, marathon runner, and then a long-course triathlete, there seemed to be a split of two camps. The resistance training (RT) athletes knew the importance of and prioritized eating protein after workouts. The endurance athletes knew they burned through large amounts of carbohydrate energy and glycogen during their prolonged training and tended to focus on eating mainly carbohydrate after workouts. We now more fully understand that all macronutrients are important for all athletes, and in my work as a sports dietician I explain both the importance of preworkout, postworkout, and overall protein intake to endurance athletes and of taking in carbohydrate to RT athletes.

Without paying attention to and meeting your recovery nutrition needs, it can take up to 72 hours after prolonged or exhaustive exercise for your body to restock its much-needed supply of muscle glycogen in your muscles (Heaton et al. 2017). Initial recovery nutrition studies showed 50 percent faster glycogen depletion when cyclists consumed 2 grams of carbohydrate per kilogram (1 g/lb) of body weight within 30 minutes after exercise versus delaying that recovery nutrition by two hours (Kerksick et al. 2017). Subsequently, in a review of many additional studies on this topic, the International

Spotlight on Paul Thompson

Paul is a two-time medalist in the World Masters Athletic Championships. He ran a 2:31.45 marathon in London in April 2017 and was the third fastest in the world that year for his age group. As luck would have it, the other two fastest runners age 50-plus in the world were also in that same race. Paul is a testament to just how well Masters athletes can continue to perform when they are able to continue to train at a high level and fuel and recover well.

What are your athletic goals now as a Masters runner?

My ultimate goal is to see if I can ever run my marathon personal record (PR) again. It is certainly unlikely but also worth aiming for. I was a semi-elite athlete at best early on, but I have managed to keep up my training and performance through my 50s. While I am not getting any faster, I am getting slower more slowly than most other people, and many others are falling off and no longer competing, so my age-graded results are continuing to improve.

How has your nutritional intake changed as a Masters runner?

The two biggest changes I have made to my diet over the years are taking in more protein and eating less sugar. I have become conscious that it is more important as I get older to make a point of getting in more protein and not just eating bread and pasta. I also weaned off sugary cereals, and instead we make our own granola with oats and a bit of honey. I have a sweet tooth and also a family history of type 2 diabetes, so my reduction in sugar intake is more general health focused than performance focused. Another thing I have changed completely is that early in my running career, in my 20s to early 30s, if the race was in the morning I wouldn't eat anything beforehand—just a cup of coffee. Of course, I know now that was not good practice, and now I certainly do eat breakfast. When I decided to continue as a Masters athlete, I realized quickly that my prerace meal was going to be key to my performance. I started to eat oatmeal and a banana or Ready Brek, which is advertised as healthy cereal for kids in the United Kingdom, two or three hours before my races. It was satisfying and nourishing, and I quickly noticed that I'd run better after eating it. The landmark event that switched my mind forever about having breakfast and fueling up was my first ever marathon. When I had just turned 40, I ran the London Marathon without eating breakfast, and you can imagine how that felt! I had an awful last 6 miles because my tank was empty. I had previously somehow been convinced that I didn't need breakfast before I ran and that my body would have adequate reserves. I suppose it did until 20 miles . . . and then it didn't. I had been aiming to be the top Masters runner in the London Marathon, and I ran the first half in 1:12, then lost five minutes in the last few miles. This triggered me to change my whole morning routine and pushed me to make time to eat breakfast and allow it to settle. Now I eat oatmeal with chia, flax seeds, and almond butter mixed in every day.

What is your prerace nutrition routine like now?

I generally eat pasta or, more recently, grain bowls the night before. There is nothing specific I need to have the night before; I just try to eat something I am confident will not upset my stomach. I will avoid anything new that I have not had before; that is my big no-no. Like many runners, I feel it is absolutely important that when I stand on the starting line I have already been to the bathroom, so I know I will not get a disrupted stomach. To accomplish this, I have my morning breakfast routine, and when I need to, I will roll on my stomach to trigger some movement, so I can go the bathroom.

Do you think about nutrition for recovery?

As I said earlier, I am confident that my nutrition is why I have been able to continue to train so much for so long. Generally speaking, I eat better now than I have ever done; I eat more consistently, more protein, and less junk, and am therefore able to have consistency in my training week in, week out, month in, month out. I am also good at listening to my body and knowing when I need to dial back when I sense that there might be an injury coming on. I can confidently say that consistency and nutrition have played the biggest roles in why I am able to continue to train and compete today. People can be set in their ways and resistant to change, but by making a few small modifications consistently over time, not with a fad diet, you just might finally be able to lose that extra couple of pounds, train smarter, and recover better. For example, if you find you are polishing off an entire bag of Doritos, next time make sure you put a bowl of grapes in front of you and know that would be much better. Making changes in your everyday life is not easy, but it does work in the long run. Speaking of Doritos, over the past few days, I managed to finish off a bag that friends left at our place over the weekend. When my friends left I had planned to send them home with the rest of the bag, but obviously I didn't end up doing that, and over a few days I finished them off. Most of the time, we don't bring those types of foods in the house. I do have a sweet tooth, but I don't need a lot of chocolate in order to satisfy my craving for something sweet. One or two Swiss Lindt chocolate balls, and I am good.

Paul's Favorite Postrace Meal

After a race, I tend to resort to normal eating almost immediately. Because most races take place early in the morning, this means I tend to have my typical weekend breakfast of, say, scrambled eggs on toast with avocado plus cereal with Greek-style yogurt.

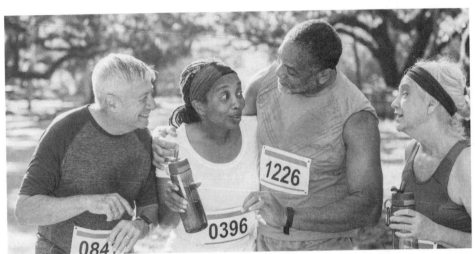

While I fully support celebrating with friends at the finish line, please also start on your recovery, too.

kali9/E+/Getty Images

Society of Sports Nutrition (ISSN) position stand recommends taking in 1.2 grams of carbohydrate per kilogram (0.5 g/lb) of body weight as soon as possible (within 30 minutes) and every 30 minutes thereafter for three and a half hours or at least 0.6 to 1.0 grams of carbohydrate as soon as possible and every two hours for four to six hours for maximum glycogen repletion (Kerksick et al. 2017). They also stress the importance of adding protein to this postexercise meal (0.2-0.4 g of protein/kg [0.1-0.2 g/lb] of body weight), especially if an athlete is unable to take in the ideal amount of carbohydrate. The American College of Sports Medicine and Academy of Nutrition and Dietitians and Dietitians of Canada joint position statement recommends the same 1.2 grams of carbohydrate per kilogram (0.5 g/lb) of body weight as soon as possible and every two hours for four to six hours or 0.8 grams of carbohydrate per kilogram (0.4 g/lb) of body weight plus 0.4 grams of protein per kilogram (0.2 g/lb) of body weight for maximum glycogen repletion and muscle protein synthesis (Thomas, Erdman, and Burke 2016). See table 13.1 for a summary of what these numbers mean for your recovery.

TABLE 13.1 Postworkout Carbohydrate Needs

	RECOMMENDATION			
Athlete weight	0.8 g of carbohydrate/kg (0.4 g/lb) of body weight	Carbohydrate calories	1.2 g of carbohydrate/kg (0.5 g/lb) of body weight	Carbohydrate calories
120 lb (54 kg)	44 g	175	65 g	262
160 (73 kg)	58 g	233	87 g	349
200 (91 kg)	73 g	291	109 g	436

All recommendations stress the fact that restoring muscle glycogen is a primary goal, and triggering muscle repair and muscle protein synthesis are of paramount long-term importance to athletes (Thomas, Erdman, and Burke 2016).

Moderate to high glycemic index (GI) carbohydrate is absorbed more quickly by our bodies and is therefore generally recommended for intake immediately after exercise, especially when time to the next session or competition is less than 72 hours, in order to increase the rate of repletion. Some examples of high GI carbohydrate are white rice, pancakes, bagels, potatoes, yogurt, smoothies, recovery drinks, and pasta (Heaton et al. 2017). Refer to table 13.2 for some typical high-carb foods (and portions) you might want to eat after workouts.

TABLE 13.2   Typical Carbohydrate Recovery Foods

Carbohydrate source	15 g carbohydrate serving size	30 g carbohydrate serving size	45 g carbohydrate serving size
Cereal (cooked)	1/2 cup	1 cup	1-1/2 cup
Pasta	1/2 cup	1 cup	1-1/2 cup
Rice	1/3 cup	2/3 cup	1 cup
Beans, lentils	1/3 cup	2/3 cup	1 cup
Pancakes	One 4" (1/4" thick) cake	Two 4" (1/4" thick) cakes	Three 4" (1/4" thick) cakes
Corn, peas	1/2 cup	1 cup	1-1/2 cup
Sweet potato	1/2 cup	1 cup	1-1/2 cup
Bagel (large)	One fourth	One half	3/4
English muffin	One half	One	1-1/2
Graham crackers	Three (2.5" squares)	Six (2.5" squares)	Nine (2.5" squares)
Apple	One small	One large	1-1/2 large
Banana (large)	One half	One	1-1/2
Berries	3/4 cup	1-1/2 cup	2-1/4 cup
Pineapple	3/4 cup	1-1/2 cup	2-1/4 cup
Cow's milk	1-1/4 cup	2-1/2 cup	3-3/4 cup
Yogurt	2/3 cup (6 oz)	1-1/2 cups (12 oz)	2-1/4 cups (18 oz)
Dried figs	One and a half	Three	Four and a half
Raisins	2 tbsp	4 tbsp	6 tbsp
Recovery drink	Varies; ~4-5 oz	Varies; ~8-10 oz	Varies; 12-16 oz

Data from Centers for Disease Control and Prevention (2020). https://www.cdc.gov/diabetes/managing/eat-well/diabetes-and-carbs/carbohydrate-choice-lists.html

While it is important to ensure adequate postworkout nutrition, it is equally as important for Masters athletes to meet their overall dietary needs and intake for total carbohydrate every day in order to fully recover and repair between sessions. Athletes with high training volumes such as back-to-back days of 85 to 90 minutes of training per day were found to fully restock glycogen within 24 hours after exhaustive exercise when they consumed more than 8 grams of carbohydrate per kilogram (4 g/lb) of body weight per day. This likely applies to a range of athletes who are training for an average of 90 minutes a day at least a few days each week at different points in their training cycle, including triathletes, soccer and rugby players, swimmers, and cyclists.

Unfortunately, during periods of repeated high-intensity training, races, or games, injury and illness rates increase, many resulting from overuse or underrecovery. Masters athletes often discuss the latest and greatest recovery tools and gadgets, including cold therapy (i.e., ice baths), cryotherapy pants and chambers; massage and home percussion massagers; compression socks, shorts, tights, and boots; rollers and trigger point therapy; TENS units; and more. While many of these tools can help our recovery, nutrition is a less expensive way to help ensure we meet our recovery needs in order to decrease our rates of illness and injury. That said, not all athletes like that high intake of carbs or find it easy to accomplish, especially without some advanced planning. See table 13.3 to help you identify your total need for daily carbohydrates.

For example, here is what a 120-pound (54 kg) athlete who is performing more than 90 minutes of exercise a day would need to consume to get in 8 grams of carbohydrate per kilogram (4 g/lb) of body weight (or 436 g of carbohydrate) per day:

- *Preworkout fuel:* one banana
- *Ninety-minute workout:* one bottle of sport drink containing 30 to 50 grams of carbohydrate
- *Postworkout recovery or breakfast:* bowl of oatmeal with fruit and honey, cottage cheese
- *Midmorning snack:* slice of pumpkin bread, yogurt
- *Lunch:* grain bowl with 1/2 cup each lentils, corn, and quinoa, plus vegetables, protein, and avocado
- *Midafternoon snack:* large apple with peanut butter
- *Dinner:* 2 cups cooked pasta with chicken, salad, two pieces of Italian bread
- *Dessert or snack:* one scoop ice cream and 1 cup berries

Getting a Preworkout Jump Start on Recovery

You might be able to start to improve your recovery even before you break a sweat. Taking in carbohydrate energy before RT sessions has been shown

TABLE 13.3 Daily Carbohydrate Needs for Masters Athletes

Recommendation	5 g of carbohydrate/kg (2 g/lb) of body weight/day	6 g of carbohydrate/kg (3 g/lb) of body weight/day	8 g of carbohydrate/kg (4 g/lb) of body weight/day	10 g of carbohydrate/kg (5 g/lb) of body weight/day
Exercise intensity and volume	Low intensity and skill based	Moderate exercise volume (about 1 hr/day)	High-volume training and competition; endurance exercise more than between 1-3 hr/day	Very high; 4-5 hr/day of moderate- to high-intensity activity
120 pound (54 kg) athlete	273 g	327 g	436 g	545 g
160 pound (73 kg) athlete	364 g	436 g	582 g	727 g
200 pound (91 kg) athlete	455 g	545 g	727 g	909 g

Data from Thomas et al. (2016).

to help decrease muscle glycogen lost during training, meaning there will be less that needs to be replenished, and your muscles will be ready to train again sooner (Kerksick et al. 2017). Additionally, taking in carbs (6% carbohydrate solution, found in a commercially available sport drink) and protein (6 g essential amino acids [EAA]) before RT has been shown to decrease cortisol levels following exercise, which may also serve to facilitate faster recovery (Kerksick et al. 2017).

Overall, exercising in a fed state (i.e., you have eaten something before you exercise) leads to decreased muscle protein breakdown and net positive amino acid balance after exercise (Aragon and Schoenfeld 2013). You owe it to your muscles to go into your workouts fueled and ready to work. To that end, studies have found that 25 grams of total protein taken before and after workouts for 14 weeks during an RT program served to increase muscle protein fiber size as well as jump height in athletes (Kerksick et al. 2017). If you are unsure of which end of the recommended range you should aim for, most Masters athletes would benefit from being at the higher end of protein intake, as long as they are also taking in adequate carbohydrate and total fat throughout the day.

By now it should be apparent that prioritizing nutrition leads to better performance and overall health. However, current research is looking at specific amounts of both carbohydrate and protein needed before, during, and after exercise in an effort to fine-tune and optimize nutritional recommendations for different athletes across sports, by gender, by training volume, and by age.

Let's turn now to Ramon Bermo, an ultra runner and coach, with whom I coached triathlon teams almost 20 years ago.

Spotlight on Ramon Bermo

Ramon Bermo, who started running as a 10-year-old growing up in Spain, has been an athlete for over 40 years. He has run more than 90 official marathons (with a PR of 2:45), 13 Ironman Triathlons including the World Championship in Kona, Hawaii (with an Ironman PR of 10:16 in 2004 at age 37), and many ultramarathons (technically defined as anything >26.2 mi, but often >50 mi). He recently completed a 240-miler and was training for a 330-mile event, The California Untamed, when we spoke for this interview. Ramon has served as the director of community development and head coach at the American Cancer Society for the past 10 years, and has coached triathletes for the New York City chapter of the Leukemia and Lymphoma Society's Team in Training (for which I also coached and where he and I met over 20 years ago), New York University athletics, and the NIKE Run Club. Ramon has dedicated his life to both his personal pursuit of sport and to helping others pursue their athletic goals.

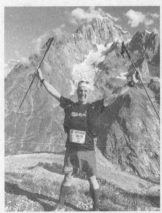

© Ramon Bermo

What nutritional changes have you made as a Masters athlete?

Did I think about nutrition 40 years ago? Are you crazy? No one was talking about nutrition. Carbo loading looked like eating as much pasta as you could the night before you ran. I started focusing on nutrition in 1997, when I did my first triathlon to celebrate my 30th birthday. By 1999 I was training for my first Ironman-branded event in the United States and started experimenting with Ensure, PB&J sandwiches, and Coca-Cola, since I knew I'd be racing for over 10 hours. I still vividly remember feeling how much it helped and that awesome feeling of cycling and running well fueled. I also remember when you and I first met, when you were giving a sport nutrition clinic to the Team in Training (TNT) triathlon team in the early 2000s. That was the first time I heard there were amounts of carbohydrate and fluid and salt I was supposed to be taking. When I first spoke with you, the amount of carbs you wanted me to take sounded so high, I thought you were crazy. Then I started adding more carbs as you suggested; I felt amazing and realized what you recommended was possible. I just hadn't practiced it before. As we get older, most athletes are more willing to do what we need to do (stretch more, eat better) because we know the consequences of not doing it. I will skip a run if I am not recovered because I don't want to miss a month if I get injured. And I make nutrition a priority so that I recover the best I can.

Here are my down-and-dirty nutritional changes as a Masters athlete:

- I pay much more attention to my recovery nutrition and never miss it no matter what.
- I eat fewer processed foods.
- I try not to eat dinner too late, which means that if I know I will not be home until ten o'clock at night, I plan in advance and eat dinner at five o'clock. Being more prepared is an adjustment that is part of continuing to run and train as a Masters athlete.

Do you have an overall nutrition philosophy?

I am from Spain, and culturally, we love eating. I have definitely shifted to eating more natural foods versus what I ate when I first moved to the United States, but I never watched everything I put in my body. I put in the work—running, cycling, and swimming—and tried to eat well. It was not realistic, nor was it necessary for me to calculate everything that I ate leading up to Ironman. I wanted to be competitive but also wanted to enjoy training and my life. It didn't make sense to me to watch my food so closely that I would no longer enjoy eating or training.

What does your fueling look like during ultra running?

For ultramarathons, I practice fueling to train my gut, and take in both sport products and real foods. Most ultra runners will tell you that at some point your body tells you it needs real foods. I have tried a hamburger or other foods that sound crazy to eat during a run, but they work because that is what my body wants. We are working at a lower heart rate/exertion rate than during a marathon, and at that level you can eat whatever your body wants. Unless we are really climbing up, then we wait. In the Tahoe 200, they offered us eggs Benedict, which I had never had before. I wasn't feeling great at that point, and tried it, plus a lemon dessert, and felt much better for the rest of the race. From then on, I realized I needed to focus on eating real foods and eating enough overall. To give you an idea, that particular event took me 83 hours. That is 83 hours of running and eating! Yesterday, I ran for 12 hours, from seven o'clock at night to seven o'clock in the morning, to practice running all night and eating while I should be sleeping. For races that allow you to have a crew, they bring you what you need. But for races when you are alone, you need to adjust. For example, I am not a chips guy, but they usually have chips at aid stations, and it actually feels good to eat these during these overnight events, so I practice what I think I will have to eat in addition to what I know I will want.

How seriously do you take your recovery nutrition?

I think it is fair to say that for most (let's say 90%) athletes I have coached over the past 24 years, posttraining nutrition is what many athletes lack. That is certainly what I focus on now and what I tell my athletes early on. We need to make sure our bodies recover well! Over the past few years I have become really informed about my postrun nutrition by literally experimenting on myself. Week one I tested how I felt when I drank chocolate milk and ate other foods within 30 minutes after each workout. After one week I could definitely tell that the effects were huge—in a very positive way. Then, just to be sure, the next week I tested only water. After that week, I saw 100 percent that the difference in my recovery is huge! You will not be surprised to hear this, but my muscles do not recover the same with water as when I take in my nutrition. This was not as noticeable when I was younger, but now it is day and night. I wish I would have learned and tried this sooner, but at least I know now. I have switched from telling my athletes to do what I say and not what I do, to really knowing I have to fuel well too and no matter how pressed for time I am, I have to do it. In the past, if I had three hours, I used to run for exactly three hours. Now I run for two and a half hours and take 30 minutes to eat and stretch.

I have been running for a long time and have had some great races, but also can't help but think that if I had been taking in proper nutrition during and after training in

> continued

> continued

those early years, I would have recovered faster, pushed harder in training, and run even faster. This is a weapon athletes now have to help them get better, that those of us old people didn't get to try out. You now have me thinking that there are many workouts I had to skip over the past 40-plus years, many of which would not have had to be missed if I had your nutritional advice to follow back then. Even though I am much older now, I can do Ironman Triathlons and more back-to-back long runs because I really focus on my nutrition. It makes all the difference.

Ramon's Favorite Postrace Meal

I love chocolate milk after workouts, but I don't think you'd consider that a meal. As a meal, definitely a big steak. The bigger and longer the event, the bigger the steak—with French fries. I want greasy and misbehaving types of food.

If Carbohydrate Is King, Protein Is Queen

Adding protein (0.2-0.4 g/kg [0.1-0.2 g/lb] of body weight/hour) to your post-workout carbohydrate intake (>0.8 g/kg [0.4 g/lb] of body weight/hour) has been shown to improve subsequent athletic performance the next morning (Kerksick et al. 2017). Overall, studies done on younger athletes show that a higher range of protein intake is required than previously thought. Ivy et al. (2002), in their early work on this topic, fed cyclists equal total calories following two and a half hours of intense cycling designed to decrease muscle glycogen stores. Their meals consisted of either 80 grams of total carbohydrate (about 1.2 g/kg [0.5 g/lb] of body weight) plus 28 grams of protein and 6 grams of fat, or 108 grams (>1.5 g/kg [0.7 g/lb] of body weight) of total carbohydrate plus 6 grams of fat 10 minutes after exercise completion and again two hours later. By four hours into recovery, muscle glycogen synthesis was significantly higher for the carbohydrate plus protein intake group.

The previously accepted amount of protein thought to be needed to maximize muscle protein synthesis after exercise was about 20 grams (0.3 g/kg [0.1 g/lb] of body weight) every three hours in addition to adequate total protein, energy, and carbohydrate over the following 24 hours to facilitate full recovery (Louis et al. 2019). Initial studies first demonstrated decreased ability to synthesize muscle protein after exercise as we age. This information inspired more studies, which have shown that higher postexercise and total daily protein intake maximize muscle protein synthesis and full recovery as we age. While 20 grams of protein may have been adequate to stimulate muscle protein synthesis in our younger days, in order to provide adequate stimulus to maintain muscle mass as we age, Masters athletes now require 35 to 40 grams of total protein after exercise and per meal (four times a day total) due to decreased anabolic sensitivity (Louis et al. 2019). This seems to be especially important for any eccentric or muscle-damaging exercise,

---

including downhill running, and for all athletes over the age of 50.

Up to 0.5 grams of protein per kilogram (0.2 g/lb) of body weight has been shown to minimize muscle protein damage, promote favorable hormone balance, and enhance recovery following intense exercise (Kerksick et al. 2017) for Masters endurance athletes as well as larger athletes and athletes looking to achieve weight loss (Louis et al. 2019). See table 13.4 for calculations on your specific recovery needs.

The ISSN position stand on nutrient timing (Kerksick et al. 2017) states that when rapid restoration or recovery time of less than four hours is required, "aggressive carbohydrate feeding" of 1.2 grams of carbohydrate per kilogram (0.5 g/lb) of body weight per hour should be considered, with a preference toward foods that are more rapidly digested or have a higher glycemic index. The alternative to this is taking in 0.8 grams of carbohydrate per kilogram (0.4 g/lb) of body weight per hour plus an additional 0.2 to 0.4 grams of protein per kilogram (0.1-0.2 g/lb) of body weight per hour. They also state that taking in carbs and protein after both RT and sport-specific or endurance training helps optimize recovery and adaptations needed before the next training session. Since dietary protein provides substrate and also acts as a trigger for muscle protein synthesis (Thomas, Erdman, and Burke 2016), this one-two protein punch has positive effects on future performance, especially when training on consecutive days or even multiple times per day (van Loon 2014).

TABLE 13.4 Postworkout Recovery Protein Needs by Body Weight

	GRAMS OF PROTEIN PER KILOGRAM OF BODY WEIGHT			
	0.2 g of protein/ kg (0.1 g/lb)	**0.3 g of protein/ kg (0.1/lb)**	**0.4 g of protein/ kg (0.2 g/lb)**	**0.5 g of protein/ kg (0.2 g/lb)**
	Minimum protein requirement immediately after exercise to help restock glycogen, especially if less than 1.2 g carbohydrate/kg is consumed	Optimal protein intake for Masters athletes as soon as possible after exercise (assuming a protein intake of a total of four or five times/ day)	Amount of protein needed (plus 0.8 g carbohydrate/ kg [0.4 g/lb]) to improve next-day performance	Amount of protein shown to minimize protein damage and enhance recovery postexercise (plus up to 1.2 g of carbohydrate/kg [0.54 g/lb]) when rapid restoration is required/desired
120-pound athlete (54 kg)	11 g	16 g	22 g	27 g
160-pound athlete (73 kg)	15 g	22 g	30 g	37 g
200-pound athlete (91 kg)	18 g	27 g	36 g	46 g

Per current research, the best sources of dietary protein for optimal recovery include EAA, specifically, rapidly absorbing leucine, which is found predominantly in dairy or whey protein. Numerous studies have found that taking in about 10 to 12 grams of EAA leads to maximum stimulation of muscle protein synthesis after exercise in younger athletes (Kerksick et al. 2017). However, 10 grams of EAA alone was not adequate to increase muscle protein synthesis in older athletes, who require 20 to 40 grams of total mixed protein. You can cover your bases and include at least 10 grams of EAA in your total of 30 to 40 grams of protein after exercise, and then include protein-rich foods three or four additional times within 24 hours (Heaton et al. 2017). Furthermore, viewing muscle protein synthesis or maintenance as a goal encourages you to consume adequate total protein within 30 minutes of completion of training sessions and competitions, as well as in your daily nutritional intake (Kerksick et al. 2017). Studies have showed that increasing Masters athletes' portions of lean meat eaten after RT exercise from about 4 ounces (about 25 g of protein) to about 6 ounces (40 g of protein) induced an increased muscle protein synthesis rate (Louis et al. 2019), and that athletes taking in a 25-gram amino acid blend (16.6 g whey protein, 2.8 g casein, 2.8 g egg, and 2 g glutamine) both before and after exercise for 14 weeks exhibited increased muscle strength and jump height (Kerksick et al. 2017). The following is an example of what a recovery-day meal plan might look like, beginning immediately after a training session, game, or race.

You can even get a jump start on your recovery before you start training or racing and help prevent muscle protein breakdown during ultraendurance exercise by including some protein in your prerace or -game meal (van Loon 2014). Luckily, it doesn't take much protein to do this; about 20 grams of intact (whole) protein or about 9 grams of EAA (leucine, isoleucine, valine) seems to do the trick (Beelen et al. 2010). And while much research (especially on younger athletes) points to specific benefits of ingesting EAA, specifically leucine, after exercise, the predominance of research on Masters athletes points to the total amount consumed both immediately after workout and throughout the day as the most important aspect of protein.

I hope this knowledge convinces you that including a pretraining yogurt, egg, serving of turkey jerky, or other protein of choice along with carbohydrate is worth the small amount of effort it takes, because it will go a long way toward your long-term success as an athlete. On the flip side, athletes who exercise in a fasted state show decreased muscle protein synthesis (Beelen et al. 2010).

To simplify your eating to meet your increasing protein needs as Masters athletes, refer to table 13.5 to give you a better idea of how much of each food you need to eat at each meal and snack in order to meet your specific protein and muscle recovery needs. You'll see that some of the serving sizes become rather large when trying to meet 40-gram protein needs; you may want to include more than one protein source per meal in order to both

Sample Recovery Nutrition Plan for High-Volume Training or Game Day

This plan was designed for a 160-pound (73 kg) athlete.

Prerace, -game, or -training fuel (6:00 a.m.)

Bagel with two eggs and fruit or other high-carb and protein combination

Training session, game, or race fuel (8:00-10:00 a.m.)

Consume 30 to 60 grams of carbohydrate/hr during the session, possibly with the addition of small amounts of protein (in the drink or snack as able)

Postworkout, -race, or -game fuel (10:30 a.m. or within 30 minutes of completion)

Consume 30 to 40 grams of protein plus 50 to 60 grams of high GI carbs in food or recovery drink (e.g., stack of pancakes, berries, whey [or vegan] protein shake made with milk of choice)

Lunch (1:00 p.m.)

Enjoy 50 to 80 grams of carbs and 30 grams of protein (e.g., sandwich on thick bread with 4 ounces of tuna filet or steak, 1 cup fruit, 1/2 to 1 cup bean and corn salad)

Snack (3:00 p.m.)

Aim for 50 to 75 grams of carbs and 20 to 30 grams of protein (e.g., large piece of fruit, 6 to 8 ounces of Greek-style yogurt, 1/4 to 1/2 cup granola

Dinner (6:00 p.m.)

Balanced meal with carbs, about 30 grams of protein, good fat, and veggies (e.g., 2 cups cooked pasta with tomato sauce or olive oil; 4 ounces of fish, chicken, or tofu; salad with avocado and olives; one slice of bread)

Snack (8:00-9:00 p.m.)

Include 40 grams of casein (from milk, yogurt, or supplement) if optimal recovery is imperative (i.e. another match, key workout, or race is within 24-48 hours), or enjoy any treat you wish.

---

reach your needs and enjoy your meal (e.g., 6 ounces of tofu and 1 to 1 1/2 cups of beans).

Studies have shown that Masters athletes, with an average age of 71, were able to increase muscle strength and quality by consuming 1.34 grams of protein per kilogram (0.61 g/lb) of body weight per day versus 1.21 grams of protein per kilogram (0.55 g/lb) of body weight per day. Especially for Masters athletes with a high training volume or who have noticed difficulty maintaining or increasing their muscle mass, if the exercise stimulus is there, this difficulty in maintaining or increasing muscle mass is likely due to decreased intake or availability of certain nutrients, overall calories, or total protein. See table 13.6 for calculations of protein recommendations per day based on body weight.

TABLE 13.5 Quality Protein Sources for Athletes

	20 g of protein	40 g of protein
Chicken breast	2.5 oz	5 oz
Fish	3 oz	6 oz
Turkey	3.5 oz	7 oz
Shrimp (large)	15 units	30 units
Tuna (canned)	3 oz	6 oz
Lean beef	3 oz	6 oz
Eggs (large)	Three whole	Six whole
Cottage cheese	7 oz	14 oz
Greek-style yogurt	7 oz	14 oz
Tofu	6 oz	12 oz
Tempeh	3.5 oz	7 oz
Chickpea pasta	2.5 oz	5 oz
Black bean pasta	2 oz	4 oz
Chickpeas	1-1/4 cup	2-1/2 cups
Edamame	1 cup	2 cups
Beans	1-1/2 cups	3 cups
Lentils	1 cup	2 cups
Red lentil pasta	2.5 oz	5 oz

Data obtained from Cronometer. www.cronometer.com.

In addition to increasing total protein needs, Masters athletes' total energy (calorie) needs must also be met, with a recommended energy availability (EA) of more than 30 kilocalories per kilogram (14 kcal/lb) of lean body mass per day to, "allow good adaptation to training and stay in good health" (Louis et al. 2019, page 50). As a sports dietitian, I am not a fan of athletes (or anyone, for that matter) counting their calorie intake for a prolonged period of time; I would rather athletes learn the science behind their needs and listen to hunger and satiety cues. However, if you are interested in calculating your needs, it can be useful to spot check whether you are meeting your total calorie, protein, carbohydrate, and fat needs periodically to ensure you are not suffering needlessly due to inadequate nutritional intake. If you are interested in getting more specific information about your resting metabolic rate (RMR) and needs, you may want to find a board-certified sports dietitian or other accredited professional to test your RMR. You can also start with this formula, where EA is energy availability, Ex EE is exercise energy expenditure, EI is energy intake (in kcals), and LBM (lean body mass) is measured in kg, if you have all of the info required to do so (Louis et al. 2019).

$$EA \text{ (kcal/kg LBM per day)} = Ex\ EE - EI/LBM$$

TABLE 13.6 Daily Protein Needs for Full Recovery in Masters Athletes

	0.8 g of protein/ kg (0.4 g/ lb) of body weight/day (RDA)	1.2 g of protein/ kg (0.5 g/ lb) of body weight/day (during low exercise periods or rest days)	1.4 g of protein/ kg (0.6 g/ lb) of body weight/ day (to maintain muscle mass)	1.6 g of protein/ kg (0.7 g/ lb) of body weight/day (for most endurance athletes)	2.0 g of protein/ kg (0.9 g/ lb) of body weight/ day (to maintain nitrogen balance with multiple daily sessions)	2.5 g of protein/ kg (1.1 g/ lb) of body weight/ day (during immobilization or rehab to boost immune function)
120 pound (54 kg) athlete	44 g	65 g	76 g	87 g	109 g	136 g
160 pound (73 kg) athlete	58 g	87 g	102 g	116 g	145 g	182 g
200 pound (91 kg) athlete	73 g	109 g	127 g	145 g	182 g	227 g

Mastering Bedtime Snacking

I have had countless conversations with athletes that begin with them asking me whether there was a time in the day after which they should not eat. Their question prompts two answers from me:

1. No, there is not.
2. If you train in the evening, you need to eat a full and complete meal afterward no matter what time it is on the clock.

Evening exercisers should note that going straight to bed without eating dinner or taking in proper recovery nutrition can be at least as bad, if not sometimes worse, than skipping your workout entirely. Regardless of what time you fit in your sweat session, recent studies show that Masters athletes may benefit from an evening (before-bed) snack that includes foods high in the slowly digesting protein casein in order to help you preserve muscle mass. Both younger and older athletes who consumed a casein-rich snack about 30 minutes before bed were found to have higher rates of muscle protein synthesis the next morning, about seven hours later (Louis et al. 2019). Casein-rich foods include dairy products such as low-fat cottage cheese, cheese, yogurt, and milk as well as casein protein powders. See table 13.7 for a list of casein-rich foods.

TABLE 13.7 High-Casein Foods for Your Bedtime Snack

High-casein foods	Serving to provide 20 grams of protein
Low-fat cottage cheese	~6 oz
Cheese	~3 oz
Greek-style yogurt	200 g (just under 1 cup)
2% cow's milk	~20 oz (2 1/2 cups)
Casein protein powder	20 g or as desired

Serving sizes rounded to nearest 0.25 ounces.

Recover From Injury

No athlete wants to discuss the prospect of getting injured and being sidelined from what we love doing, but every athlete has to recovery from injury, surgery, or illness at one time or another. When this happens, they often come to me concerned about how much fitness they might lose and weight they might gain but aren't initially as concerned about what they need to be eating to help optimize their recovery and minimize muscles mass loss during such times.

All athletes will lose muscle mass any time a limb needs to be immobilized, but we Masters will lose it faster. To combat some of this undesirable loss of muscle size and strength, you should prioritize adequate protein intake, specifically the amino acid leucine, during this crucial recovery time. Most athletes will find that a good-quality, third party–tested protein supplement will help them meet their needs during this phase of muscle maintenance (Holm et al. 2006). Look for one that contains 15 to 30 grams of total protein (or consume one at a rate of more than 0.4 g of protein/kg [0.2 g/lb] of body weight), and aim for taking in a serving of quality protein with every meal or snack, every three to four hours (Louis et al. 2019).

Consuming 10 grams of creatine monohydrate daily for two weeks followed by consuming 5 grams of creatine monohydrate plus 3 grams of HMB (beta-hydroxy-beta-methylbutyrate, a metabolite of the EAA leucine) daily was shown to promote muscle protein synthesis and help prevent muscle catabolism during immobilization and rehabilitation as well as meet increased protein needs for recovery (Louis et al. 2019).

Role of Fluids

As you well know by now, staying hydrated is extremely important to both performance and recovery for all athletes. This is especially true for athletes who train or compete in the heat, perform indoors without adequate ventilation, wear heavy equipment, and do twice-daily sessions or long sessions on back-to-back days.

You hopefully also remember that sodium is the key electrolyte lost in sweat that needs to be replaced in order to maintain the body's delicate fluid balance. Sodium is also an important regulator of thirst, so including sodium in your postworkout fluid or foods is paramount to optimizing your rehydration quickly (Heaton et al. 2017). Plain water can be a great overall hydrator through our normal, busy days, but drinking plain water without intake of salty food after workouts will only cause our drive to drink to shut down prior to full restoration of our body's hydration status. Therefore, it is important to choose a rehydration beverage that contains sodium (about 20-50 mmol/L) or ensure you have salty foods (e.g., pickles, tomato juice, soup) with your early recovery meal or snack (Heaton et al. 2017), especially since most athletes finish their sessions at a fluid deficit that needs to be replenished in order for the body to fully recover (Thomas, Erdman, and Burke 2016). Aim to drink 1.25 to 1.5 liters of sodium-containing fluid (or water plus salty foods) for each kilogram of body weight lost to sweat during any training session, game, or race, because fluid losses continue to occur during the cool-down and recovery phases (Heaton et al. 2017; Thomas, Erdman, and Burke 2016).

Most athletes find that chilled beverages and those with added flavor and sodium increase their drive to drink and promote better voluntary rehydration (i.e., without having to calculate your fluid needs after each session). Alcohol intake should be minimized during early recovery since it acts a diuretic and will only serve to further dehydrate you during this key time (Thomas, Erdman, and Burke 2016).

Additional Recovery Nutrition Tips and Tricks

Beyond what we've already discussed at length, we have a few other ways to aid recovery.

Omega-3 Fatty Acids

Omega-3 fats, or polyunsaturated fatty acids (PUFA) as we affectionately call them, are needed for cell membrane production, nervous system function, blood pressure regulation, glucose tolerance, and cell signaling processes, and to decrease the inflammatory processes in our bodies (Heaton et al. 2017). You may have heard recommendations of omega-3 fat supplementation to decrease risk of heart disease, some cancers, and arthritis symptoms due to its ability to decrease inflammation in the body. As such, and since intense exercise is known to increase inflammation and damage seen in our cells, studies have also looked at the benefits of supplementing athletes with two specific omega-3 fats: Eicosapentaenoic acid (EPA) and docosahexaenoic acid (DHA). These important fats are found in cold-water fatty fish (including salmon and tuna), krill oil, and fish oil supplements, but are not often consumed in large enough quantity or with adequate frequency in the typical diet to maximize their full potential. Flax, canola, soy, pumpkin seeds, and walnuts, all vegetarian sources of these healthy fats, contain another PUFA, Alpha-linolenic acid (ALA), which can be converted to EPA or DHA in our bodies (Gammone et al. 2018).

More studies are still needed, but recent studies have found that taking 2 to 4 grams of fish oil per day for eight weeks may help increase muscle building in athletes following an RT program as long as it is also accompanied by adequate total protein intake (Louis et al. 2019). Some studies have demonstrated increases in both strength and functional capacity in adults of all ages with the addition of a fish oil supplement. Others show decreases in self-reported muscle soreness ratings after eccentric exercise. Still others have demonstrated increases in immune function following six weeks of omega-3 supplementation after exercise and a lower incidence of upper-respiratory infections following supplementation during a 16-week training block (Heaton et al. 2017). Other studies have shown that a six-month period of supplementation of 3.2 grams of EPA plus 2.0 grams of DHA per day led to increased muscle strength in older people, and that supplementation with omega-3 increased thigh measurements, hamstring strength, and 1 repetition max, and helped to prevent the decline in muscle mass normally seen in adults ages 60 to 85 (Gammone et al. 2018).

Optimal dosages have not yet been determined, and there is evidence to support the benefit of decreasing DOMS for a wide range of intake, from 1.8 to 3.0 grams a day (Ranchordas, Dawson, and Russell 2017).

Caution: Athletes who have a history of bleeding, are currently taking anticoagulant drugs or supplements, or are at an increased risk of bleeding for any reason should not take high doses of fish oil without consulting their physician due to increased risk of bleeding when taking an omega-3 supplement (Mayo Clinic 2020b).

Creatine Monohydrate

Creatine is a non-EAA that is produced in the liver, pancreas, and kidneys and can also be obtained in our diet, mainly from meat, poultry, and fish (Heaton et al. 2017). Creatine has been associated with decreased inflammation and increased glycogen resynthesis, and is known to help support training adaptations. Studies have suggested that taking a creatine supplement in addition to ingesting adequate carbohydrate after exercise can improve postexercise glycogen resynthesis and increase fat-free mass and strength (Heaton et al. 2017). Supplementation with 20 grams of creatine per day for five days before exercise followed by a daily maintenance dose of 5 grams has been shown to increase muscle creatine stores by 20 percent and maintain higher creatine stores. This could be an important difference, especially for athletes whose sports are heavily dependent on creatine and phosphocreatine such as high-intensity, short-duration sports including weightlifting and sprinting.

During repeated soccer games, phosphocreatine stores are known to diminish significantly due to the frequent high-intensity activity required at high-level play (Ranchordas, Dawson, and Russell 2017). Studies have demonstrated similar benefits in soccer players taking 5 grams of creatine monohydrate four times per day for five to seven days, then a maintenance dose of 3 to 5 grams daily, or in those players taking about 3 grams a day for 28 consecutive days, in terms of helping increase phosphocreatine stores and muscle glycogen repletion. Current research suggests that creatine supplementation can benefit players when taken prior to major competitions and tournaments. Its use about 90 minutes prior to the start of a game may also help counteract the negative effects commonly seen due to sleep deficits experienced by athletes prior to major competitions (due to nerves, travel, time change, etc.). It may also help athletes who require accuracy in skills such as passing and throwing outperform their sleep-deprived peers by 20 percent, comparable to the benefits seen when athletes ingest caffeine (at 1-5 mg/kg [1-2 mg/lb] of body weight) at that same interval (Ranchordas, Dawson, and Russell 2017).

Caffeine

Most athletes will be happy to hear caffeine may not just be for your usual preworkout energy and motivation boost any longer. Recent studies have shown that adding caffeine to your postexercise carbohydrate intake (1.2 g/kg [0.5 g/lb] of body weight) may serve to further boost glycogen resynthesis following exercise (Ranchordas, Dawson, and Russell 2017). This postexercise nutritional protocol also leads to improvements in subsequent high-intensity interval run training.

Studies in elite soccer players have shown that 4 to 8 milligrams of caffeine per kilogram (2-4 mg/lb) of body weight taken after games led to higher glycogen resynthesis four hours later. This finding is especially important for all athletes who need to perform again rapidly (Ranchordas, Dawson, and Russell 2017). Beelen et al. (2010) studied cyclists and found that adding caffeine and protein to necessary carbohydrate after glycogen-depleting cycling helped athletes restore muscle glycogen synthesis faster over the subsequent four-hour recovery period. They suggested that a much more reasonable 2 milligrams of caffeine per kilogram (1 mg/lb) of body weight added to 1.0 gram of carbohydrate per kilogram (0.5 g/lb) of body weight may be the lowest effective dose. Lourerio et al. (2018) analyzed many recent studies on caffeine for recovery and concluded that caffeine can help increase insulin sensitivity and glycogen synthesis, as long as carbohydrate intake is also adequate during the recovery window.

An important note here is that doses of caffeine used in these studies were high—generally, 8 milligrams of caffeine per kilogram (4 mg/lb) of body weight. For a 120-pound (54 kg) athlete, this comes to 430 grams, or more than 30 ounces of coffee. This level is both impractical and ill-advised for most athletes due to the high risk of unwanted side effects. For reference, although everyone's caffeine tolerance is individual, 400 milligrams daily has been set as a safe upper limit. Above that limit, you risk jitteriness, anxiety, migraine headaches, restlessness, nervousness, rapid heart rate, stomach upset, and, of course, an inability to sleep if caffeine is consumed later in the day (Mayo Clinic 2020a). There is more research to be done, but in the meantime, please go ahead and enjoy your favorite caffeinated drink after your workout, race, or match without guilt and with hope of subsequent performance benefits. Aim for 2 mg/kg (or 0.9 mg/lb) of body weight, which is just over 100 mg for a 120-pound athlete, or approximately 8 ounces of coffee.

Vitamin D

Vitamin D plays many important roles in our bodies, including supporting muscle repair and recovery. If you are lucky enough to be working out outside, in the sunlight, below the 35th parallel latitude, your body should be continually making adequate vitamin D, as it was designed to. For those of us who live in the northern hemisphere, who train early or late in the day, or who wear sunblock, our bodies will not be able to produce enough vitamin D.

Low vitamin D status of active individuals has been significantly correlated with both acute and long-term muscle weakness following intense exercise (Heaton et al. 2017), as well as slower reaction time, poor balance, and higher fall risk (Ogan and Pritchett 2013). Vitamin D is a key factor in preventing stress fractures and maintaining optimal bone health (Ogan and Pritchett 2013). The Institute of Medicine's recommendation for individuals ages 1 to 70 is to take 600 IU of vitamin D daily. If your level is found to be deficient (per a lab test your primary care doctor can run for you), you can make an effort to increase your intake of fatty fish, egg yolks, and vitamin D–fortified foods. Supplementation at 800 IU vitamin D/day in older adults has been shown to increase strength and distance covered, while 5,000 IU of vitamin D for eight weeks was shown to increase vitamin D status from 11.62 to 41.27, which not only returned that lab value to normal range, but also served to increase sprint time and vertical jump. Athletes at the highest level may require as much as 3,000-5,000 IU of vitamin D daily to meet their increased needs. (Ogan and Pritchett 2013).

Antioxidants

Strenuous exercise increases oxidative stress on the body, but exercise also upregulates the body's antioxidant production, which increases a natural repair of oxidative damage (Heaton et al. 2017). For the past several decades, many athletes have taken antioxidants. However, recent studies show that chronic and high-dose supplementation of antioxidants including vitamins C and E may negatively affect the body's natural adaptations to training and are therefore not generally recommended (Ranchordas, Dawson, and Russell 2017). Eating a diet rich in fruits and vegetables, however, can more naturally boost your antioxidant intake and not surprisingly, has never been shown to negatively affect important training adaptations. The only times I, as a board-certified sports dietitian, might recommend antioxidant supplementation to athletes is during an intense and short-term competition phase (e.g., cycling stage race or weekend soccer or tennis tournament), when training responses are not warranted but short-term recovery is paramount (Heaton et al. 2017; Ranchordas, Dawson, and Russell 2017).

Beetroot, Tart Cherry Juice, and Black Tea Extract

While antioxidant supplementation is generally not recommended after training or long term, studies have shown decreases in DOMS when 500 milliliters (18 oz) of tart cherry juice was ingested by semiprofessional soccer players after games (Ranchordas, Dawson, and Russell 2017). In marathon runners drinking 355 milliliters (12 oz) of tart cherry juice daily for five days prior to and two days after running a marathon has been found to decrease muscle damage, inflammation, and oxidative stress 48 hours after completing this strenuous event (Howatson et al. 2010). They found that total antioxidant status increased after ingestion of tart cherry juice and served to aid muscle recovery, decrease markers of inflammation, and decrease perceived muscle soreness compared to a placebo. Other studies have showed similar and promising results in team-sport athletes. Some, but not all, studies on taking beetroot juice after exercise have shown promising results in terms of decreased muscle soreness. However, more research is needed regarding intake or supplementation of high-antioxidant juices and fruits, omega-3-rich foods or supplements, and more to determine specific guidelines by sport and age to both maximize training adaptations and reduce inflammation after exercise.

Since we know the importance of adequate carbohydrate intake after exercise, and many athletes report difficulty either eating after strenuous exercise or taking in adequate total carbohydrate through their busy and tiring training and racing days, taking in some of those much-needed carbs in the form of tart cherry juice might be worth a try before and after your next big race.

Enriched black tea extract has also been shown to increase recovery and decrease both oxidative stress and muscle soreness following back-to-back sessions (Ranchordas, Dawson, and Russell 2017). This aligns with other recent findings that caffeine intake after exercise helps to restock muscle glycogen faster.

In this book, you have heard from many inspiring Masters athletes; learned about the most recent studies on sport nutrition; and read nutrition blueprints for your training, races or competitions, and recovery. As you continue to train hard, you are now armed with the information you need to fully fuel, fully recover, and truly benefit from whatever activities you choose to pursue. And as you do, please feel free to reach out to me to tell me your nutritional trials and triumphs and ask me questions along the way.

REFERENCES

Chapter 1

American Heart Association. 2020. "How Much Sugar Is Too Much?" Accessed May 6, 2020. www.heart.org/en/healthy-living/healthy-eating/eat-smart/sugar/how-much-sugar-is-too-much.

Blanck, H.M., C. Gillespie, J.E. Kimmons, J.D. Seymour, and M.K Serdula. 2008. "Trends in Fruit and Vegetable Consumption Among U.S. Men and Women, 1994–2005." *Preventing Chronic Disease* 5 (2): A35.

Dietary Guidelines Advisory Committee. 2015. *Scientific Report of the 2015 Dietary Guidelines Advisory Committee: Advisory Report to the Secretary of Health and Human Services and the Secretary of Agriculture*. U.S. Department of Agriculture, Agricultural Research Service, Washington, DC. Accessed March 15, 2019. https://health.gov/sites/default/files/2019-09/Scientific-Report-of-the-2015-Dietary-Guidelines-Advisory-Committee.pdf.

Fédération Internationale de Natation (FINA). 2019. "Overview and History." Accessed March 15, 2019. www.fina.org/content/fina-aquatics-bit-history.

Masters Football League. 2020. "Masters Football League." Accessed March 15, 2019. www.mastersfootballleague.leaguerepublic.com.

MastersHistory.org. 2020. "A History of Masters Track and Field 1968 to 1971." Accessed September 6, 2020. Last modified August 16, 2020 by the Masters Track and Field History Sub-Committee. http://mastershistory.org/a-history-of-masters-track-and-field-1968-to-1971.

Masters Swimming Canada. 2020. "About Masters Swimming Canada." Accessed March 10, 2019. www.mastersswimmingcanada.ca/WP/en/aboutus/.

National Senior Games Association. 2020. "History of the NSGA." Accessed September 6, 2020. https://nsga.com/history.

NPR, Robert Wood Johnson Foundation, and Harvard T.H. Chan School of Public Health. 2015. "Sports and Health in America." Accessed March 15, 2019. https://media.npr.org/documents/2015/june/sportsandhealthpoll.pdf.

United Premier Soccer League. 2019. "UPSL Masters." Accessed March 15, 2019. www.upslsoccer.com/masters.

U.S. Department of Agriculture. 2020. "Choose My Plate." Accessed May 6, 2020. www.choosemyplate.gov/.

U.S. Department of Health and Human Services. 2017. "Only 1 in 10 Adults Get Enough Fruits or Vegetables." Last modified November 16, 2017. www.cdc.gov/media/releases/2017/p1116-fruit-vegetable-consumption.html.

U.S. Department of Health and Human Services and U.S. Department of Agriculture. 2015a. "Shifts Needed to Align with Healthy Eating Patterns." *2015-2020 Dietary Guidelines for Americans*, 8th edition. Accessed May 6, 2020. www.health.gov/our-work/food-nutrition/2015-2020-dietary-guidelines/guidelines/chapter-2/current-eating-patterns-in-the-united-states.

U.S. Department of Health and Human Services and U.S. Department of Agriculture. 2015b. *2015-2020 Dietary Guidelines for Americans*, 8th edition. Accessed March 16, 2019. www.health.gov/dietaryguidelines/2015/guidelines.

U.S. Food and Drug Administration. 2016. "You May Be Surprised by How Much Salt You're Eating." Accessed May 6, 2020. www.fda.gov/consumers/consumer-updates/you-may-be-surprised-how-much-salt-youre-eating.

U.S. Masters Swimming. 2020. "What Is U.S. Masters Swimming?" Accessed March 15, 2019. www.usms.org/about-usms/what-is-us-masters-swimming.

World Health Organization. 2020. "Healthy Diet." Accessed May 6, 2020. www.who.int/news-room/fact-sheets/detail/healthy-diet.

Worldometer. 2020. "United States Population." Accessed April 27, 2020. www.worldometers.info/world-population/us-population/.

Zong, G., A. Gao, F.B. Hu, and Q. Sun. 2016. "Whole Grain Intake and Mortality From All Causes, Cardiovascular Disease, and Cancer A Meta-Analysis of Prospective Cohort Studies." *Circulation* 133: 2370-2380. https://doi.org/10.1161/CIRCULATIONAHA.115.021101.

Chapter 2

Andrade, A., G.G. Bevilacqua, D.R. Coimbra, F.S. Pereira, and R. Brandt. 2016. "Sleep Quality, Mood and Performance: A Study of Elite Brazilian Volleyball Athletes." *Journal of Sports Science and Medicine* 15 (4): 601-605.

Boss, G.R., and J.E. Seegmiller. 1981. "Age-Related Physiological Changes and Their Clinical Significance." *Western Journal of Medicine* 135 (6): 434-440.

Campbell, W.W., M.C. Crim, V.R. Young, and W.J. Evans. 1994. "Increased Energy Requirements and Changes in Body Composition with Resistance Training in Older Adults." *American Journal of Clinical Nutrition* 60 (2): 167-175.

Chalé, A., G.J. Cloutier, C. Hau, E.M. Phillips, G.E. Dallal, and R.A. Fielding. 2012. "Efficacy of Whey Protein Supplementation on Resistance Exercise–Induced Changes in Lean Mass, Muscle Strength, and Physical Function in Mobility-Limited Older Adults." *Journals of Gerontology: Series A* 68 (6): 682-690.

Edwards, B., D. Odriscoll, A. Ali, A. Jordan, J. Trinder, and A. Malhotra. 2010. "Aging and Sleep: Physiology and Pathophysiology." *Seminars in Respiratory and Critical Care Medicine* 31 (5): 618-633.

Farage, M.A., K.W. Miller, P. Elsner, and H.I. Maibach. 2013. "Characteristics of the Aging Skin." *Advances in Wound Care* 2 (1): 5-10.

Halson, S.L. 2014. "Sleep in Elite Athletes and Nutritional Interventions to Enhance Sleep." *Sports Medicine* 44 (S1): 13-23.

Hansen, A.L., L. Dahl, G. Olson, D. Thorton, I.E. Graff, L. Frøyland, J.F. Thayer, and S. Pallesen. 2014. "Fish Consumption, Sleep, Daily Functioning, and Heart Rate Variability." *Journal of Clinical Sleep Medicine* 10 (5): 567-575.

Holick, M.F. 1996. "Vitamin D and Bone Health." *Journal of Nutrition* April 126 (S4): 1159S-1164S. https://doi.org/10.1093/jn/126.suppl_4.1159S.

Holick, M.F., N.C. Binkley, H.A. Bischoff-Ferrari, C.M. Gordon, D.A. Hanley, R.P. Heaney, M.H. Murad, and C.M. Weaver. 2011. "Evaluation, Treatment, and Prevention of Vitamin D Deficiency: An Endocrine Society Clinical Practice Guideline." *Journal of Clinical Endocrinology and Metabolism* 96 (7): 1911-1930.

Institute of Medicine, Food and Nutrition Board. 2010. *Dietary Reference Intakes for Calcium and Vitamin D.* Accessed May 4, 2020. Washington, DC: The National Academy Press. www.nap.edu/read/13050/chapter/24.

Kalapotharakos, V.I., K. Diamantopoulos, and S.P. Tokmakidis. 2010. "Effects of Resistance Training and Detraining on Muscle Strength and Functional Performance of Older Adults Aged 80 to 88 Years." *Aging Clinical and Experimental Research* 22 (2): 134-140.

Kim, J.Y., J.K. Paik, O.Y. Kim, H.W. Park, J.H. Lee, Y. Jang, and J.H. Lee. 2011. "Effects of Lycopene Supplementation on Oxidative Stress and Markers of Endothelial Function in Healthy Men." *Atherosclerosis* 215 (1): 189-195.

Landowne, M., M. Brandfonbrener, and N.W. Shock. 1955. "The Relation of Age to Certain Measures of Performance of the Heart and the Circulation." *Circulation* 12 (4): 567-576.

Lundholm, K., G. Holm, L. Lindmark, B. Larsson, L. Sjöström, and P. Björntorp. 1986. "Thermogenic Effect of Food in Physically Well-Trained Elderly Men." *European Journal of Applied Physiology and Occupational Physiology* 55 (5): 486-492.

National Osteoporosis Foundation. 2020. "Bone Health Basics: Get the Facts." Accessed April 13, 2020. www.nof.org/prevention/general-facts.

National Sleep Foundation. 2003. "2003 Sleep and Aging." Accessed August 9, 2020. www.sleepfoundation.org/professionals/sleep-americar-polls/2003-sleep-and-aging.

National Sleep Foundation. 2019. "Menopause and Sleep." Accessed April 14, 2019. www.sleepfoundation.org/articles/menopause-and-sleep.

National Sleep Foundation. 2020. "Foods to Eat for a Good Night's Sleep." Accessed May 14, 2020. www.sleep.org/articles/foods-for-sleep.

Pollock, M.L., C. Foster, D. Knapp, J.L. Rod, and D.H. Schmidt. 1987. "Effect of Age and Training on Aerobic Capacity and Body Composition of Master Athletes." *Journal of Applied Physiology* 62 (2): 725-731.

Pradhan, G., S.L. Samson, and Y. Sun. 2013. "Ghrelin: Much More Than a Hunger Hormone." *Current Opinion in Clinical Nutrition and Metabolic Care* 16 (6): 619-624.

Schagen, S.K., V.A. Zampeli, E. Makrantonaki, and C.C. Zouboulis. 2012. "Discovering the Link Between Nutrition and Skin Aging." *Dermato-Endocrinology* 4 (3): 298-307.

Short, K.R., J.L. Vittone, M.L. Bigelow, D.N. Proctor, and K.S. Nair. 2004. "Age and Aerobic Exercise Training Effects on Whole Body and Muscle Protein Metabolism." *American Journal of Physiology-Endocrinology and Metabolism* 286 (1): E92-E101.

Strasser, B., K. Volaklis, D. Fuchs, and M. Burtscher. 2018. "Role of Dietary Protein and Muscular Fitness on Longevity and Aging." *Aging and Disease* 9 (1): 119-132.

Swann, J.B., and M.J. Smyth. 2007. "Immune Surveillance of Tumors." *Journal of Clinical Investigation* 117 (5): 1137-1146.

Tanaka, H., and D.R. Seals. 2003. "Invited Review: Dynamic Exercise Performance in Masters Athletes: Insight into the Effects of Primary Human Aging on Physiological Functional Capacity." *Journal of Applied Physiology* 95 (5): 2152-2162.

Tzellos, T.G., I. Klagas, K. Vahtsevanos, S. Triaridis, A. Printza, A. Kyrgidis, G. Karakiulakis, C.C. Zouboulis, and E. Papakonstantinou. 2009. "Extrinsic Ageing in the Human Skin Is Associated With Alterations in the Expression of Hyaluronic Acid and Its Metabolizing Enzymes." *Experimental Dermatology* 18 (12): 1028-1035.

Van Cauter, E., K. Spiegel, E. Tasali, and R. Leproult. 2008. "Metabolic Consequences of Sleep and Sleep Loss." *Sleep Medicine* 9 (S1): S23-S28.

Chapter 3

Agarwal, S.K. 2012. "Cardiovascular Benefits of Exercise." *International Journal of General Medicine* 5: 541-545.

Amati, F., J.J. Dube, P.M. Coen, M. Stefanovic-Racic, F.G. Toledo, and B.H. Goodpaster. 2009. "Physical Inactivity and Obesity Underlie the Insulin Resistance of Aging." *Diabetes Care* 32 (8): 1547-1549.

American Cancer Society. 2019. "Cancer Facts & Figures 2019." Accessed May 8, 2020.

www.cancer.org/research/cancer-facts-statistics/all-cancer-facts-figures/cancer-facts-figures-2019.html.

American College of Sports Medicine (ACSM), W.J. Chodzko-Zajko, D.N. Proctor, M.A. Fiatarone Singh, C.T. Minson, C.R. Nigg, G.J. Salem, and J.S. Skinner. 2009. "American College of Sports Medicine Position Stand. Exercise and Physical Activity for Older Adults." *Medicine and Science in Sports and Exercise* 41 (7): 1510-1530.

American Diabetes Association. 2018. "Statistics About Diabetes." Accessed May 8, 2020. www.diabetes.org/resources/statistics/statistics-about-diabetes.

Benjamin, E.J., P. Muntner, A. Alonso, M.S. Bittencourt, C.W. Callaway, A.P. Carson, A.M. Chamberlain, A.R. Chang, S. Cheng, S.R. Das, F.N. Delling, L. Djousee, M.S.V. Elkind, J.F. Ferguson, M. Fornage, L. Chaffin Jordan, S.S. Khan, B.M. Kissela, K.L. Knutson, T.W. Kwan, D.T. Lackland, T.T. Lewis, J.H. Lichtman, C.T. Longnecker, M.S. Loop, P.L. Lutsey, S.S. Martin, K. Matsushita, A.E. Moran, M.E. Mussolino, M. O'Flaherty, A. Pandey, A.M. Perak, W.D. Rosamond, G.A. Roth, U.K.A. Sampson, G.M. Satou, E.B. Schroeder, S.H. Shah, N.L. Spartano, A. Stokes, D.L. Tirschwell, C.W. Tsao, M.P. Turakhia, L.B. VanWagner, J.T. Wilkins, S.S. Wong, S.S. Virani, and American Heart Association Council on Epidemiology and Prevention Statistics Committee and Stroke Statistics Subcommittee. 2019. "Heart Disease and Stroke Statistics—2019 Update: A Report from the American Heart Association." *Circulation* 139 (10): e56-e528.

Centers for Disease Control and Prevention (CDC). 2019a. "What Is Diabetes?" Accessed December 15, 2019. www.cdc.gov/diabetes/basics/diabetes.html.

Centers for Disease Control and Prevention (CDC). 2019b. "Heart Disease Facts." Accessed May 8, 2020. www.cdc.gov/heartdisease/facts.htm.

Gudmundsdottir, H., A. Høieggen, A, Stenehjem, B. Waldum, and I. Os. 2012. "Hypertension in Women: Latest Findings and Clinical Implications." *Therapeutic Advances in Chronic Disease* 3 (3): 137-146.

Hoy, M.K., and J.D. Goldman. 2014. "Fiber Intake of the U.S. Population: What We Eat in America, NHANES 2009-2010." Food Surveys Research Group, Dietary Data Brief No. 12, September 2014. Accessed September 6, 2020. https://www.ars.usda.gov/ARSUserFiles/80400530/pdf/DBrief/12_fiber_intake_0910.pdf.

Maas, A.H.E.M., and Y.E.A. Appelman. 2010. "Gender Differences in Coronary Heart Disease." *Netherlands Heart Journal* 18 (12): 598-602.

Mozaffarian, D., T. Hao, E.B. Rimm, W.C. Willett, and F.B. Hu. 2011. "Changes in Diet and Lifestyle and Long-Term Weight Gain in Women and Men." *New England Journal of Medicine* 364 (25): 2392-2404.

Oldways Whole Grains Council. 2019. "Whole Grains 101." Accessed December 16, 2019. www.wholegrainscouncil.org/whole-grains-101.

Reynolds, A., J. Mann, J. Cummings, N. Winter, E. Mete, and L. Te Morenga. 2019. "Carbohydrate Quality and Human Health: A Series of Systematic Reviews and Meta-Analyses." *Lancet* 393 (10170): 434-445.

Whelton, P.K., R.M. Carey, W.S. Aronow, D.E. Casey Jr., K.J. Collins, C. Dennison Himmelfarb, S.M. DePalma, S. Gidding, K.A. Jamerson, D.W. Jones, E.J. MacLaughlin, P. Muntner, B. Ovbiagele, S.C. Smith Jr., C.C. Spencer, R.S. Stafford, S.J. Taler, R.J. Thomas, K.A. Williams Sr., J.D. Williamson, and J.T. Wright Jr. 2018. "2017 ACC/AHA/AAPA/ABC/ACPM/AGS/APhA/ASH/ASPC/NMA/PCNA Guideline for the Prevention, Detection, Evaluation, and Management of High Blood Pressure in Adults: A Report of the American College of Cardiology/American Heart Association Task Force on Clinical Practice Guidelines." *Journal of the American College of Cardiology* 71 (19): e127-e248.

Chapter 4

Harvard School of Public Health. 2011. "The Best Diet: Quality Counts." Accessed December 6, 2019. www.hsph.harvard.edu/nutritionsource/healthy-weight/best-diet-quality-counts/.

Kerksick, C.M., S. Arent, B.J. Schoenfeld, J.R. Stout, B. Campbell, C.D. Wilborn, L. Taylor, D. Kalman, A.E. Smith-Ryan, R.B. Kreider, D. Willoughby, P.J. Arciero, T.A. VanDusseldorp, M.J. Ormsbee, R. Wildman, M. Greenwood, T.N. Ziegenfuss, A.A. Aragon, and J. Antonio. 2017. "International Society of Sports Nutrition Position Stand: Nutrient Timing." *Journal of the International Society of Sports Nutrition* 14: 33. https://doi.org/10.1186/s12970-017-0189-4.

Larsen, T.M., S.M. Dalskov, M. van Baak, S.A. Jebb, A. Papadaki, A.F.H. Pfeiffer, J.A. Martinez, T. Handjieva-Darlenska, M. Kunešová, M. Philsgård, S. Stender, and C. Holst. 2010. "Diets With High or Low Protein Content and Glycemic Index for Weight-Loss Maintenance." *New England Journal of Medicine* 363 (22): 2102-2113. https://doi.org/10.1056/NEJMoa1007137.

Mozaffarian, D., T. Hao, E.B. Rimm, W.C. Willett, and F.B. Hu. 2011. "Changes in Diet and Lifestyle and Long-Term Weight Gain in Women and Men." *New England Journal of Medicine* 364 (25): 2392-2404. https://doi.org/10.1056/NEJMoa1014296.

Sacks, F.M., G.A. Bray, V.J. Carey, S.R. Smith, D.H. Ryan, S.D. Anton, K. McManus, C.M. Champagne, L.M. Bishop, N. Laranjo, M.S. Leboff, J.C. Rood, L. de Jonge, F.L. Greenway, C.M. Loria, E. Obarzanek, and D.A. Williamson. 2009. "Comparison of Weight-Loss Diets With Different Compositions of Fat, Protein, and Carbohydrates." *New England Journal of Medicine* 360 (9): 859-873. https://doi.org/10.1056/NEJMoa0804748.

Chapter 5

Achten, J., S.L. Halson, L. Moseley, M.P. Rayson, A. Casey, and A.E. Jeukendrup. 2004. "Higher Dietary Carbohydrate Content During Intensified Running Training Results in Better Maintenance of Performance and Mood State." *Journal of Applied Physiology* 96 (4): 1331-1340.

Bartlett, J.D., J.A. Hawley, and J.P. Morton. 2015. "Carbohydrate Availability and Exercise Training Adaptation: Too Much of a Good Thing?" *European Journal of Sport Science* 15 (1): 3-12.

Burke, L.M., J.A. Hawley, S.H.S. Wong, and A.E. Jeukendrup. 2011. "Carbohydrates for Training and Competition." *Journal of Sports Sciences* 29 (S1): S17-S27.

Doering, T., P. Reaburn, N. Borges, and D. Jenkins. 2015. "Low Carbohydrate Intake of Masters vs. Young Triathletes in the Pre-Competition Phase of Training." *Journal of Science and Medicine in Sport* 19: e91. https://doi.org/10.1016/j.jsams.2015.12.353.

Dubé, J.J., N.T. Broskey, A.A. Despines, M. Stefanovic-Racic, F.G. Toledo, B.H. Goodpaster, and F. Amati. 2016. "Muscle Characteristics and Substrate Energetics in Lifelong Endurance Athletes." *Medicine and Science in Sports and Exercise* 48 (3): 472-480.

Jacobs, K.A., and W.M. Sherman. 1999. "The Efficacy of Carbohydrate Supplementation and Chronic High-Carbohydrate Diets for Improving Endurance Performance." *International Journal of Sport Nutrition and Exercise Metabolism* 9 (1): 92-115.

Kanter, M. 2018. "High-Quality Carbohydrates and Physical Performance." *Nutrition Today* 53 (1): 35-39.

Lane, S.C., J.L. Areta, S.R. Bird, V.G. Coffey, L.M. Burke, B. Desbrow, L.G. Karagounis, and J.A. Hawley. 2013. "Caffeine Ingestion and Cycling Power Output in a Low or Normal Muscle Glycogen State." *Medicine and Science in Sports and Exercise* 45 (8): 1577-1584.

Melzer, K. 2011. "Carbohydrate and Fat Utilization During Rest and Physical Activity."

E-SPEN 6 (2): e45-e52.

Ormsbee, M.J., C.W. Bach, and D.A. Baur. 2014. "Pre-Exercise Nutrition: The Role of Macronutrients, Modified Starches and Supplements on Metabolism and Endurance Performance." *Nutrients* 6 (5): 1782-1808.

Stepto, N.K, A.L Carey, H.M. Staudacher, N.K. Cummings, L.M. Burke, and J.A. Hawley. 2002. "Effect of Short-Term Fat Adaptation on High-Intensity Training." *Medicine and Science in Sports and Exercise* 34 (3): 449-455.

Thomas, D.T., K.A. Erdman, and L.M. Burke. 2016. "Position of the Academy of Nutrition and Dietetics, Dietitians of Canada, and the American College of Sports Medicine: Nutrition and Athletic Performance." *Journal of the Academy of Nutrition and Dietetics* 116 (3): 501-528.

Chapter 6

Breen, L., and S.M. Phillips. 2011. "Skeletal Muscle Protein Metabolism in the Elderly: Interventions to Counteract the Anabolic Resistance of Ageing." *Nutrition and Metabolism* 8: 68.

Burke, L.M., L.M. Castell, D.J. Casa, G.L. Close, R.J.S. Costa, B. Desbrow, S.L. Halson, D.M. Lis, A.K. Melin, P. Peeling, P.U. Saunders, G.J. Slater, J. Sygo, O.C. Witard, S. Bermon, and T. Stellingwerff. 2019. "International Association of Athletics Federations Consensus Statement 2019: Nutrition for Athletics." *International Journal of Sport Nutrition and Exercise Metabolism* 29 (2): 73-84.

Cermak, N.M., P.T. Res, L.C.P.G.M. de Groot, W.H.M. Saris, and L.J.C. van Loon. 2012. "Protein Supplementation Augments the Adaptive Response of Skeletal Muscle to Resistance-Type Exercise Training: A Meta-Analysis." *American Journal of Clinical Nutrition* 96 (6): 1454-1464.

Knuiman, P., M.T.E. Hopman, C. Verbruggen, and M. Mensink. 2018. "Protein and the Adaptive Response With Endurance Training: Wishful Thinking or a Competitive Edge?" *Frontiers in Physiology* 9: 598.

Koopman, R., D.L.E. Pannemans, A.E. Jeukendrup, A.P. Gijsen, J.M.G. Senden, D. Halliday, W.H.M. Saris, L.J.C. Van Loon, and A.J.M. Wagenmakers. 2004. "Combined Ingestion of Protein and Carbohydrate Improves Protein Balance During Ultra-Endurance Exercise." *American Journal of Physiology-Endocrinology and Metabolism* 287 (4): E712-E720.

Moore, D.R., T.A. Churchward-Venne, O. Witard, L. Breen, N.A. Burd, K.D. Tipton, and S.M. Phillips. 2014. "Protein Ingestion to Stimulate Myofibrillar Protein Synthesis Requires Greater Relative Protein Intakes in Healthy Older Versus Younger Men." *Journals of Gerontology Series A* 70 (1): 57-62.

Phillips, B.E., P.J. Atherton, K. Varadhan, M.C. Limb, D.J. Wilkinson, K.A. Sjøberg, K. Smith, and J.P. Williams. 2015. "The Effects of Resistance Exercise Training on Macro- and Micro-Circulatory Responses to Feeding and Skeletal Muscle Protein Anabolism in Older Men." *Journal of Physiology* 593 (12): 2721-2734.

Phillips, S.M. 2011. "The Science of Muscle Hypertrophy: Making Dietary Protein Count." *Proceedings of the Nutrition Society* 70 (1): 100-103.

Strasser, B., K. Volaklis, D. Fuchs, and M. Burtscher. 2018. "Role of Dietary Protein and Muscular Fitness on Longevity and Aging." *Aging and Disease* 9 (1): 119-132.

Tarnopolsky, M.A. 2008. "Nutritional Consideration in the Aging Athlete." *Clinical Journal of Sport Medicine* 18 (6): 531-538.

Thomas, D.T., K.A. Erdman, and L.M. Burke. 2016. "Position of the Academy of Nutrition and Dietetics, Dietitians of Canada, and the American College of Sports Medicine: Nutrition and Athletic Performance." *Journal of the Academy of Nutrition and Dietetics* 116

(3): 501-528.

Tipton, K.D., B.B. Rasmussen, S.L. Miller, S.E. Wolf, S.K. Owens-Stovall, B.E. Petrini, and R.R. Wolfe. 2001. "Timing of Amino Acid-Carbohydrate Ingestion Alters Anabolic Response of Muscle to Resistance Exercise." *American Journal of Physiology-Endocrinology and Metabolism* 281 (2): E197-E206.

Van Loon, L.J. 2014. "Is There a Need for Protein Ingestion During Exercise?" *Sports Medicine* 44 (Suppl 1): 105-111.

Volpi, E., H. Kobayashi, M. Sheffield-Moore, B. Mittendorfer, and R.R. Wolfe. 2003. "Essential Amino Acids Are Primarily Responsible for the Amino Acid Stimulation of Muscle Protein Anabolism in Healthy Elderly Adults." *American Journal of Clinical Nutrition* 78 (2): 250-258.

Chapter 7

American Heart Association. 2017. "The American Heart Association Diet and Lifestyle Recommendations." Accessed March 11, 2020. www.heart.org/en/healthy-living/healthy-eating/eat-smart/nutrition-basics/aha-diet-and-lifestyle-recommendations.

Bartlett, J.D., J.A. Hawley, and J.P. Morton. 2015. "Carbohydrate Availability and Exercise Training Adaptation: Too Much of a Good Thing?" *European Journal of Sport Science* 15 (1): 3-12.

Burke, L.M., D.J. Angus, G.R. Cox, N.K. Cummings, M.A. Febbraio, K. Gawthorn, J.A. Hawley, M. Minehan, D.T. Martin, and M. Hargreaves. 2000. "Effect of Fat Adaptation and Carbohydrate Restoration on Metabolism and Performance During Prolonged Cycling." *Journal of Applied Physiology* 89 (6): 2413-2421.

Goldman, T.R. 2016. "Health Policy Brief: Final 2015–2020 Dietary Guidelines for Americans." *Health Affairs*, March 31, 2016.

Gordon, B. 2019. "Choose Healthy Fats." Accessed March 12, 2020. www.eatright.org/food/nutrition/dietary-guidelines-and-myplate/choose-healthy-fats.

Kerksick, C.M., C.D. Wilborn, M.D. Roberts, A. Smith-Ryan, S.M. Kleiner, R. Jäger, R. Collins, M. Cooke, J.N. Davis, E. Galvan, M. Greenwood, L.M. Lowery, R. Wildman, J. Antonio, and R.B. Kreider. 2018. "ISSN Exercise and Sports Nutrition Review Update: Research and Recommendations." *Journal of the International Society of Sports Nutrition* 15 (1): 38.

Liu, A.G., N.A. Ford, F.B. Hu, K.M. Zelman, D. Mozaffarian, and P.M. Kris-Etherton. 2017. "A Healthy Approach to Dietary Fats: Understanding the Science and Taking Action to Reduce Consumer Confusion." *Nutrition Journal* 16 (1): 53.

Thomas, D.T., K.A. Erdman, and L.M. Burke. 2016. "Position of the Academy of Nutrition and Dietetics, Dietitians of Canada, and the American College of Sports Medicine: Nutrition and Athletic Performance." *Journal of the Academy of Nutrition and Dietetics* 116 (3): 501-528.

Tiller, N.B., J.D. Roberts, L. Beasley, S. Chapman, J.M. Pinto, L. Smith, M. Wiffin, M. Russell, S.A. Sparks, L. Duckworth, J. O'Hara, L. Sutton, J. Antonio, D.S. Willoughby, M.D. Tarpey, A.E. Smith-Ryan, M.J. Ormsbee, T.A. Astorino, R.B. Kreider, G.R. McGinnis, J.R. Stout, J.W. Smith, S.M. Arent, B.I. Campbell, and L. Bannock. 2019. "International Society of Sports Nutrition Position Stand: Nutritional Considerations for Single-Stage Ultra-Marathon Training and Racing." *Journal of the International Society of Sports Nutrition* 16 (1): 50.

Chapter 8

Anderson, M.E., C.R. Bruce, S.F. Fraser, N.K. Stepto, R. Klein, W.G. Hopkins, and J.A. Hawley. 2000. "Improved 2000-Meter Rowing Performance in Competitive Oarswomen

After Caffeine Ingestion." *International Journal of Sport Nutrition and Exercise Metabolism* 10 (4): 464-475.

Attele, A.S., J.T. Xie, and C.S. Yuan. 2000. "Treatment of Insomnia: An Alternative Approach." *Alternative Medicine Review* 5 (3): 249-259.

Butts, J., B. Jacobs, and M. Silvis. 2017. "Creatine Use in Sports." *Sports Health: A Multidisciplinary Approach* 10 (1): 31-34.

Centers for Disease Control and Prevention (CDC). 2019. "Faststats: Osteoporosis." Accessed November 1, 2019. www.cdc.gov/nchs/fastats/osteoporosis.htm.

Christensen, P.M., Y. Shirai, C. Ritz, and N.B. Nordsborg. 2017. "Caffeine and Bicarbonate for Speed. A Meta-Analysis of Legal Supplements Potential for Improving Intense Endurance Exercise Performance." *Frontiers in Physiology* 8: 240.

Cinosi, E., G. Di Iorio, T. Acciavatti, M. Cornelio, F. Vellante, L. De Risio, and G. Martinotti. 2011. "Sleep Disturbances in Eating Disorders: A Review." *Clinical Therapeutics* 162 (6): e195-e202.

Clark, K.L., W. Sebastianelli, K.R. Flechsenhar, D.F. Aukermann, F. Meza, R.L. Millard, J.R. Deitch, P.S. Sherbondy, and A. Albert. 2008. "24-Week Study on the Use of Collagen Hydrolysate as a Dietary Supplement in Athletes With Activity-Related Joint Pain." *Current Medical Research and Opinion* 24 (5): 1485-1496.

Council for Responsible Nutrition (CRN). 2019. "Dietary Supplement Use Reaches All-Time High—Available-for-Purchase Consumer Survey Reaffirms the Vital Role Supplementation Plays in the Lives of Most Americans." Accessed November 1, 2019. www.crnusa.org/CRNConsumerSurvey#top.

Domínguez, R., J.L. Maté-Muñoz, E. Cuenca, P. García-Fernández, F. Mata-Ordoñez, M.C. Lozano-Estevan, P. Veiga-Herreros, S.F. da Silva, and M.V. Garnacho-Castaño. 2018. "Effects of Beetroot Juice Supplementation on Intermittent High-Intensity Exercise Efforts." *Journal of the International Society of Sports Nutrition* 15: 2. https://doi.org/10.1186/s12970-017-0204-9.

Gibson, R.S. 2005. *Principles of Nutritional Assessment.* 2nd edition. New York: Oxford University Press.

Grgic, J., I. Grgic, C. Pickering, B.J. Schoenfeld, D.J. Bishop, and Z. Pedisic. 2019. "Wake Up and Smell the Coffee: Caffeine Supplementation and Exercise Performance—An Umbrella Review of 21 Published Meta-Analyses." *British Journal of Sports Medicine* 54: 681-688.

Hadzic, M., M.L. Eckstein, and M. Schugardt. 2019. "The Impact of Sodium Bicarbonate on Performance in Response to Exercise Duration in Athletes: A Systemic Review." *Journal of Sports Science and Medicine* 18: 271-281.

Halson, S.L. 2014. "Sleep in Elite Athletes and Nutritional Interventions to Enhance Sleep." *Sports Medicine* 44 (S1): 13-23.

Hewlings, S., and D. Kalman. 2017. "Curcumin: A Review of Its Effects on Human Health." *Foods* 6 (10): 92. https://doi.org/10.3390/foods6100092.

Juszkiewicz, A., A. Glapa, P. Basta, E. Petriczko, K. Z.ołnowski, B. Machalin'ski, J. Trzeciak, K. Łuczkowska, and A. Skarpan'ska-Stejnborn. 2019. "The Effect of L-Theanine Supplementation on the Immune System of Athletes Exposed to Strenuous Physical Exercise." *Journal of the International Society of Sports Nutrition* 16 (1): 7.

Kaufman, C. 2018. "Foods to Fight Iron Deficiency." Accessed November 1, 2019. www.eatright.org/health/wellness/preventing-illness/iron-deficiency.

Kuehl, K.S, E.T. Perrier, D.L. Elliot, and J.C. Chesnutt. 2010. "Efficacy of Tart Cherry Juice in Reducing Muscle Pain During Running: A Randomized Controlled Trial." *Journal of the International Society of Sports Nutrition* 7: 17.

Kunstel, K. 2005. "Calcium Requirements for the Athlete." *Current Sports Medicine Reports* 4 (4): 203-206.

Lane, J.D., J.F. Steege, S.L. Rupp, and C.M. Kuhn. 1992. "Menstrual Cycle Effects on Caffeine Elimination in the Human Female." *European Journal of Clinical Pharmacology* 43 (5): 543-546.

Latunde-Dada, G.O. 2012. "Iron Metabolism in Athletes—Achieving a Gold Standard." *European Journal of Haematology* 90 (1): 10-15.

López-Flores, M., R.L. Nieto, O.C. Moreira, D.S. Iglesias, and J.G. Villa. 2018. "Effects of Melatonin on Sports Performance: A Systematic Review." *Journal of Exercise Physiology Online* 21 (5): 121-138.

Maughan, R.J., L.M. Burke, J. Dvorak, D.E. Larson-Meyer, P. Peeling, S.M. Phillips, E.S. Rawson, N.P. Walsh, I. Garthe, H. Geyer, R. Meeusen, L.J.C. van Loon, S.M. Shirreffs, L.L. Spriet, M. Stuart, A. Vernec, K. Currell, V.M. Ali, R.G. Budgett, A. Ljungqvist, M. Mountjoy, Y.P. Pitsiladis, T. Soligard, U. Erdener, and L. Engebretsen. 2018. "IOC Consensus Statement: Dietary Supplements and the High-Performance Athlete." *British Journal of Sports Medicine* 52 (7): 439-455.

National Institutes of Health (NIH), Office of Dietary Supplements. 2019. "Calcium: Fact Sheet for Health Professionals." Accessed November 1, 2019. https://ods.od.nih.gov/factsheets/Calcium-HealthProfessional/.

Nehlig, A. 2018. "Interindividual Differences in Caffeine Metabolism and Factors Driving Caffeine Consumption." *Pharmacological Reviews* 70 (2): 384-411.

Saunders, B., K. Elliott-Sale, G.G. Artioli, P.A. Swinton, E. Dolan, H. Roschel, C. Sale, and B. Gualano. 2017. "B-Alanine Supplementation to Improve Exercise Capacity and Performance: A Systematic Review and Meta-Analysis." *British Journal of Sports Medicine* 51 (8): 658-669.

Tallis, J., M.J. Duncan, S. Leddington Wright, E.L.J. Eyre, E. Bryant, D. Langdon, and R.S. James. 2013. "Assessment of the Ergogenic Effect of Caffeine Supplementation on Mood, Anticipation Timing, and Muscular Strength in Older Adults." *Physiological Reports* 1 (3): e00072.

Taylor, L., B.C.R. Chrismas, B. Dascombe, K. Chamari, and P.M. Fowler. 2016. "Sleep Medication and Athletic Performance—The Evidence for Practitioners and Future Research Directions." *Frontiers in Physiology* 7: 83. https://doi.org/10.3389/fphys.2016.00083.

Tromp, M.D., A.A. Donners, J. Garssen, and J.C. Verster. 2016. "Sleep, Eating Disorder Symptoms, and Daytime Functioning." *Nature and Science of Sleep* 8: 35-40.

Vitale, K.C., S. Hueglin, and E. Broad. 2017. "Tart Cherry Juice in Athletes." *Current Sports Medicine Reports* 16 (4): 230-239.

Williams, M.H. 2004. "Dietary Supplements and Sports Performance: Introduction and Vitamins." *Journal of the International Society of Sports Nutrition* 1 (2): 1-6.

Chapter 9

American College of Sports Medicine (ACSM), M.N. Sawka, L.M. Burke, E.R. Eichner, R.J. Maughan, S.J. Montain, and N.J. Stachenfeld. 2007. "American College of Sports Medicine Position Stand. Exercise and Fluid Replacement." *Medicine and Science in Sports and Exercise* 39 (2): 377-390.

Baker, L.B., and A.E. Jeukendrup. 2014. "Optimal Composition of Fluid-Replacement Beverages." *Comprehensive Physiology* 4 (2): 575-620.

Balmain, B.N., S. Sabapathy, M. Louis, and N.R. Morris. 2018. "Aging and Thermoregulatory

Control: The Clinical Implications of Exercising Under Heat Stress in Older Individuals." *BioMed Research International.* https://doi.org/10.1155/2018/8306154.

Guyton, A.C, and J.E. Hall. 2000. *Textbook of Medical Physiology.* 10th edition. Philadelphia: W.B. Saunders.

Institute of Medicine (IOM). 2005. *Dietary Reference Intakes for Water, Potassium, Sodium, Chloride, and Sulfate.* Washington, DC: The National Academies Press.

LaFata, D., A. Carlson-Phillips, S.T. Sims, and E.M. Russell. 2012. "The Effect of a Cold Beverage During an Exercise Session Combining Both Strength and energy Systems Development Training on Core Temperature and Markers of Performance." *Journal of the International Society of Sports Nutrition* 9 (1): 44. https://doi.org/10.1186/1550-2783-9-44.

Logan-Sprenger, H.M., G.J. Heigenhauser, K.J. Killian, and L.L. Spriet. 2012. "Effects of Dehydration During Cycling on Skeletal Muscle Metabolism in Females." *Medicine and Science in Sports and Exercise* 44 (10): 1949-1957.

Logan-Sprenger, H.M., G.J. Heigenhauser, G.L. Jones, and L.L. Spriet. 2015. "The Effect of Dehydration on Muscle Metabolism and Time Trial Performance During Prolonged Cycling in Males." *Physiological Reports* 3 (8): e12483. https://doi.org/10.14814/phy2.12483.

Maughan, R.J., and S.M. Shirreffs. 2008. "Development of Individual Hydration Strategies for Athletes." *International Journal of Sport Nutrition and Exercise Metabolism* 18 (5): 457-472.

Maughan, R.J., and S.M. Shirreffs. 2010. "Dehydration and Rehydration in Competitive Sport." *Scandinavian Journal of Medicine and Science in Sports* 20 (April): 40-47.

Sawka, M.N. 1992. "Physiological Consequences of Hypohydration: Exercise Performance and Thermoregulation." *Medicine and Science in Sports and Exercise* 24 (6): 657-670.

Sawka, M.N., S.N. Cheuvront, and R.W. Kenefick. 2015. "Hypohydration and Human Performance: Impact of Environment and Physiological Mechanisms." *Sports Medicine* 45 (S1): 51-60.

Shirreffs, S.M., A.J. Taylor, J.B. Leiper, and R.J. Maughan. 1996. "Post-Exercise Rehydration in Man: Effects of Volume Consumed and Drink Sodium Content." *Medicine and Science in Sports and Exercise* 28 (10): 1260-1271.

Thomas, D.T., K.A. Erdman, and L.M. Burke. 2016. "Position of the Academy of Nutrition and Dietetics, Dietitians of Canada, and the American College of Sports Medicine: Nutrition and Athletic Performance." *Journal of the Academy of Nutrition and Dietetics* 116 (3): 501-528.

Walter, A.N., and T.L. Lenz. 2011. "Hydration and Medication Use." *American Journal of Lifestyle Medicine* 5 (4): 332-335.

Chapter 10

Bär, K.-J., and V. Markser. 2013. "Sport Specificity of Mental Disorders: The Issue of Sport Psychiatry." *European Archives of Psychiatry and Clinical Neuroscience* 263 (Suppl 2): S205-S210.

Gibbs, J.C., N.I. Williams, and M.J. De Souza. 2013. "Prevalence of Individual and Combined Components of the Female Athlete Triad." *Medicine and Science in Sports and Exercise* 45 (5): 985-996.

Hausenblas, H.A., and D.S. Downs. 2002. *Exercise Dependence Scale-21 Manual.* http://www.personal.psu.edu/dsd11/EDS/EDS21Manual.pdf.

Keay, N., G. Francis, and K. Hind. 2018. "Low Energy Availability Assessed by a Sport-Specific Questionnaire and Clinical Interview Indicative of Bone Health, Endocrine Profile and Cycling Performance in Competitive Male Cyclists." *BMJ Open Sport and Exercise*

Medicine 4 (1): e000424. https://doi.org/10.1136/bmjsem-2018-000424.

Mehta, J., B. Thompson, and J.M. Kling. 2018. "The Female Athlete Triad: It Takes a Team." *Cleveland Clinic Journal of Medicine* 85 (4): 313-320.

Mountjoy, M., J. Sundgot-Borgen, L. Burke, K.E. Ackerman, C. Blauwet, N. Constantini, C. Lebrun, B. Lundy, A. Melin, N. Meyer, R. Sherman, A.S. Tenforde, M.K. Torstveit, and R. Budgett. 2018. "International Olympic Committee (IOC) Consensus Statement on Relative Energy Deficiency in Sport (RED-S): 2018 Update." *International Journal of Sport Nutrition and Exercise Metabolism* 28 (4): 316-331.

National Eating Disorders Association (NEDA). 2018. "Statistics and Research on Eating Disorders." Accessed on June 26, 2020. https://www.nationaleatingdisorders.org/statistics-research-eating-disorders.

Nattiv, A., A.B. Loucks, M.M. Manore, C.F. Sanborn, J. Sundgot-Borgen, M.P. Warren, and American College of Sports Medicine. 2007. "American College of Sports Medicine Position Stand. The Female Athlete Triad." *Medicine and Science in Sports and Exercise* 39 (10): 1867-1882.

Otis, C.L., B. Drinkwater, M. Johnson, A. Loucks, and J. Wilmore. 1997. "American College of Sports Medicine Position Stand. The Female Athlete Triad." *Medicine and Science in Sports and Exercise* 29 (5): i-ix.

Payne, J.M., and J.T. Kitchener. 2014. "Should You Suspect the Female Athlete Triad?" *Journal of Family Practice* 63: 187-192.

Sardar, M.R., A. Greway, M. DeAngelis, E.O. Tysko, S. Lehmann, M. Wohlstetter, and R. Patel. 2015. "Cardiovascular Impact of Eating Disorders in Adults: A Single Center Experience and Literature Review." *Heart Views* 16 (3): 88-92.

Thein-Nissenbaum, J. 2013. "Long-Term Consequences of the Female Athlete Triad." *Maturitas* 75 (2): 107-112.

Torstveit, M.K., I.L. Fahrenholtz, M.B. Lichtenstein, T.B. Stenqvist, and A.K. Melin. 2019. "Exercise Dependence, Eating Disorder Symptoms and Biomarkers of Relative Energy Deficiency in Sports (RED-S) Among Male Endurance Athletes." *BMJ Open Sport and Exercise Medicine* 5 (1): e000439. https://doi.org/10.1136/bmjsem-2018-000439.

Vanheest, J.L., C.D. Rodgers, C.E. Mahoney, and M.J. De Souza. 2014. "Ovarian Suppression Impairs Sport Performance in Junior Elite Female Swimmers." *Medicine and Science in Sports and Exercise* 46 (1): 156-166.

Chapter 11

Bartlett, J.D., J.A. Hawley, and J.P. Morton. 2015. "Carbohydrate Availability and Exercise Training Adaptation: Too Much of a Good Thing?" *European Journal of Sport Science* 15 (1): 3-12.

Burke, L.M., J.A. Hawley, S.H.S. Wong, and A.E. Jeukendrup. 2011. "Carbohydrates for Training and Competition." *Journal of Sports Sciences* 29 (Suppl 1): S17-S27.

Bussau, V.A., T.J. Fairchild, A. Rao, P. Steele, and P.A. Fournier. 2002. "Carbohydrate Loading in Human Muscle: An Improved 1 Day Protocol." *European Journal of Applied Physiology* 87 (3): 290-295.

Close, G.L., K. Baar, C. Sale, and S. Bermon. 2019. "Nutrition for the Prevention and Treatment of Injuries in Track and Field Athletes." *International Journal of Sport Nutrition and Exercise Metabolism* 29 (2): 189-197.

Jeukendrup, A.E., and S. Killer. 2010. "The Myths Surrounding Pre-Exercise Carbohydrate Feeding." *Annals of Nutrition and Metabolism* 57 (Suppl 2): 18-25.

Oliver, J.M., A.L. Almada, L.E. Van Eck, M. Shah, J.B. Mitchell, M.T. Jones, A.R. Jagim, and D.S. Rowlands. 2016. "Ingestion of High Molecular Weight Carbohydrate Enhances Subsequent Repeated Maximal Power: A Randomized Controlled Trial." *PLOS ONE* 11 (9): 1-17.

Ormsbee, M.J., C.W. Bach, and D.A. Baur. 2014. "Pre-Exercise Nutrition: The Role of Macronutrients, Modified Starches and Supplements on Metabolism and Endurance Performance." *Nutrients* 6 (5): 1782-1808.

Thomas, D.T., K.A. Erdman, and L.M. Burke. 2016. "Position of the Academy of Nutrition and Dietetics, Dietitians of Canada, and the American College of Sports Medicine: Nutrition and Athletic Performance." *Journal of the Academy of Nutrition and Dietetics* 116 (3): 501-528.

Chapter 12

Baltazar-Martins, G., and J. Del Coso. 2019. "Carbohydrate Mouth Rinse Decreases Time to Complete a Simulated Cycling Time Trial." *Frontiers in Nutrition* 6: 65.

Burke, L.M., J.A. Hailey, S.H.S. Wong, and A.E. Jeukendrup. 2011. "Carbohydrate for Training and Competition." *Journal of Sports Science* 29 (S1): S17-S27.

Jeukendrup, A. 2014. "A Step Towards Personalized Sports Nutrition: Carbohydrate Intake During Exercise." *Sports Medicine* 44 (S1): 25-33.

Kerksick, C.M., S. Arent, B.J. Schoenfeld, J.R. Stout, B. Campbell, C.D. Wilborn, L. Taylor, D. Kalman, A.E. Smith-Ryan, R.B. Kreider, D. Willoughby, P.J. Arciero, T.A. VanDusseldorp, M.J. Ormsbee, R. Wildman, M. Greenwood, T.N. Ziegenfuss, A.A. Aragon, and J. Antonio. 2017. "International Society of Sports Nutrition Position Stand: Nutrient Timing." *Journal of the International Society of Sports Nutrition* 14: 33.

Kimber, N.E., J.J. Ross, S.L. Mason, and D.B. Speedy. 2002. "Energy Balance During an Ironman Triathlon in Male and Female Triathletes." *International Journal of Sport Nutrition and Exercise Metabolism* 12 (1): 47-62.

Ormsbee, M., C. Bach, and D. Baur. 2014. "Pre-Exercise Nutrition: The Role of Macronutrients, Modified Starches and Supplements on Metabolism and Endurance Performance." *Nutrients* 6 (5): 1782-1808.

Thomas, D.T., K.A. Erdman, and L.M. Burke. 2016. "Position of the Academy of Nutrition and Dietetics, Dietitians of Canada, and the American College of Sports Medicine: Nutrition and Athletic Performance." *Journal of the Academy of Nutrition and Dietetics* 116 (3): 501-528.

Viribay, A., S. Arribalzaga, J. Mielgo-Ayuso, A. Castañeda-Babarro, J. Seco-Calvo, and A. Urdampilleta. 2020. "Effects of 120 g/h of Carbohydrate Intake During a Mountain Marathon on Exercise-Induced Muscle Damage in Elite Runners." *Nutrients* 12 (5): 1367.

Chapter 13

Aragon, A.A., and J. Schoenfeld. 2013. "Nutrient Timing Revisited: Is There a Post-Exercise Anabolic Window?" *Journal of the International Society of Sports Nutrition* 10 (1): 5.

Beelen, M., L.M. Burke, M.J. Gibala, and L.J.C. van Loon. 2010. "Nutritional Strategies to Promote Postexercise Recovery." *International Journal of Sport Nutrition and Exercise Metabolism* 20 (6): 515-532.

Gammone, M., G. Riccioni, G. Parrinello, and N. D'Orazio. 2018. "Omega-3 Polyunsaturated Fatty Acids: Benefits and Endpoints in Sport." *Nutrients* 11 (1): 46.

Gray, W. 2019. "Want to Know All About This Month's IRONMAN World Championship in Kailua-Kona, Hawai'i? Check Out These Stunning Stats on the People, Places and Performances That Make It So Special." *Redbull.* Last modified October 1, 2019. https://www.redbull.com/us-en/kona-ironman-stats.

Heaton, L.E., J.K. Davis, E.S. Rawson, R.P. Nuccio, O.C. Witard, K.W. Stein, K. Baar, J.M. Carter, and L.B. Baker. 2017. "Selected In-Season Nutritional Strategies to Enhance Recovery for Team Sport Athletes: A Practical Overview." *Sports Medicine* 47 (11): 2201-2218.

Holm, L., B. Esmarck, M. Mizuno, H. Hansen, C. Suetta, P. Hölmich, M. Krogsgaard, and M. Kjær. 2006. "The Effect of Protein and Carbohydrate Supplementation on Strength Training Outcome of Rehabilitation in ACL Patients." *Journal of Orthopaedic Research* 24 (11): 2114-2123.

Howatson, G., M.P. McHugh, J.A. Hill, J. Brouner, A.P. Jewell, K.A. Van Someren, R.E. Shave, and S.A. Howatson. 2010. "Influence of Tart Cherry Juice on Indices of Recovery Following Marathon Running." *Scandinavian Journal of Medicine and Science in Sports* 20 (6): 843-852.

Ivy, J.L., H.W. Goforth, B.M. Damon, T.R. McCauley, E.C. Parsons, and T.B. Price. 2002. "Early Postexercise Muscle Glycogen Recovery Is Enhanced With a Carbohydrate-Protein Supplement." *Journal of Applied Physiology* 93 (4): 1337-1344.

Kerksick, C.M., S. Arent, B.J. Schoenfeld, J.R. Stout, B. Campbell, C.D. Wilborn, L. Taylor, D. Kalman, A.E. Smith-Ryan, R.B. Kreider, D. Willoughby, P.J. Arciero, T.A. VanDusseldorp, M.J. Ormsbee, R. Wildman, M. Greenwood, T.N. Ziegenfuss, A.A. Aragon, and J. Antonio. 2017. "International Society of Sports Nutrition Position Stand: Nutrient Timing." *Journal of the International Society of Sports Nutrition* 14: 33.

Louis, J., F. Vercruyssen, O. Dupuy, and T. Bernard. 2019. "Nutrition for Master Athletes: From Challenges to Optimisation Strategies." *Movement and Sport Sciences (Science et Motricité)* 104: 45-54.

Loureiro, L.M.R., C.E. Gonçalves Reis, and T.H. Macedo Da Costa. 2018. "Effects of Coffee Components on Muscle Glycogen Recovery: A Systematic Review." *International Journal of Sport Nutrition and Exercise Metabolism* 28 (3): 284-293.

Mayo Clinic. 2020a. "Drugs and Supplements: Caffeine (Oral Route). Side Effects." Accessed on January 18, 2020. www.mayoclinic.org/drugs-supplements/caffeine-oral-route/side-effects/drg-20137844.

Mayo Clinic. 2020b. "Fish Oil. Overview." Accessed February 18, 2020. www.mayoclinic.org/drugs-supplements-fish-oil/art-20364810.

Ogan, D., and K. Pritchett. 2013. "Vitamin D and the Athlete: Risks, Recommendations, and Benefits." *Nutrients* 5 (6): 1856-1868. https://doi.org/10.3390/nu5061856.

Ranchordas, M.K., J.T. Dawson, and M. Russell. 2017. "Practical Nutritional Recovery Strategies for Elite Soccer Players When Limited Time Separates Repeated Matches." *Journal of the International Society of Sports Nutrition* 14: 35.

Thomas, D.T., K.A. Erdman, and L.M. Burke. 2016. "American College of Sports Medicine Joint Position Statement: Nutrition and Athletic Performance." *Medicine and Science in Sports and Exercise* 48 (3): 543-568.

van Loon, L.J.C. 2014. "Is There a Need for Protein Ingestion During Exercise?" *Sports Medicine* 44 (S1): 105-111.

INDEX

Note: Page references followed by an italic *f* or *t* indicate information contained in figures or tables, respectively.

ABOUT THE AUTHOR

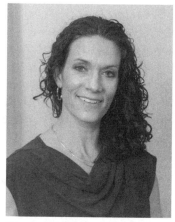

© Lauren Antonucci

Lauren A. Antonucci, MS, RDN, CSSD, CDE, CDN, is the owner and director of Nutrition Energy, where she creates individualized plans that fit the lifestyle of each client, helps them develop a healthy relationship with food and their bodies, and guides them to reach their nutrition and health goals. She is a registered dietitian nutritionist (RDN), is certified by the Academy of Nutrition and Dietetics as a specialist in sports dietetics (CSSD), and is certified by the National Certification Board for Diabetes Educators as a diabetes educator (CDE).

Antonucci has been running, swimming, and cycling for as long as she can remember and has completed 13 marathons (PR 3:09), three Ironman Triathlons, and countless other running and triathlon races. She is a sought-after presenter on the topic of sport nutrition and hydration, and she has presented at many professional conferences, including American College of Sports Medicine (ACSM), USA Triathlon International Coaching Symposium, the Greater New York Dietetic Association (GNYDA), and many New York Road Runners (NYRR) events and New York City Marathon Expos. She has also presented to numerous collegiate athletic teams, most running and triathlon teams and clubs in New York City, and many corporate organizations.

Antonucci wrote a nutrition column for *Triathlete* magazine for three years and wrote for *New York Road Runners* magazine for over a decade. She has appeared on several television programs to provide practical advice on a wide array of nutrition and health topics, and her advice has also been featured in *Runner's World*, Ironmanlive.com, NYTimes.com, *Diabetes Self-Management*, *Time Out New York*, *Metrosports*, and many other publications.

She earned a bachelor's degree in psychobiology from Binghamton University, was awarded a fellowship in nutritional biochemistry at the University of California at Berkeley, and earned a master's degree in clinical nutrition from New York University. She lives in New York City with her husband and three children and is a proud Masters athlete.

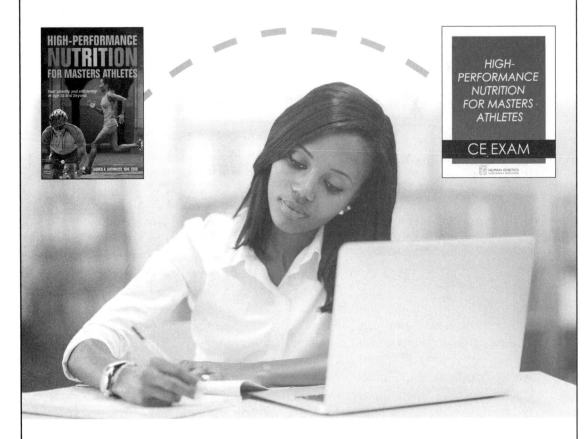
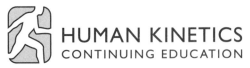